Food and Nutrition

Food and Nutrition

Customs and culture

Second edition

Paul Fieldhouse
Health Promotion Specialist
Manitoba Ministry of Health
Canada

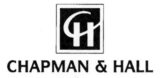

CHAPMAN & HALL

London · Glasgow · Weinheim · New York · Tokyo · Melbourne · Madras

Published by Chapman & Hall, 2–6 Boundary Row, London SE1 8HN, UK

Chapman & Hall, 2–6 Boundary Row, London SE1 8HN, UK

Blackie Academic & Professional, Wester Cleddens Road, Bishopbriggs, Glasgow G64 2NZ, UK

Chapman & Hall GmbH, Pappelallee 3, 69469 Weinheim, Germany

Chapman & Hall USA, 115 Fifth Avenue, New York, NY 10113, USA

Chapman & Hall Japan, ITP-Japan, Kyowa Building, 3F, 2-2-1 Hirakawacho, Chiyoda-ku, Tokyo 102, Japan

Chapman & Hall Australia, 102 Dodds Street, South Melbourne, Victoria 3205, Australia

Chapman & Hall India, R. Seshadri, 32 Second Main Road, CIT East, Madras 600 035, India

Distributed in the USA and Canada by Singular Publishing Group Inc., 4284 41st Street, San Diego, California 92105

First edition 1985

Reprinted 1990, 1992 and 1993

Second edition 1995

© 1985, 1995 Paul Fieldhouse

Typeset in 10/12pt Palatino by Saxon Graphics Ltd, Derby
Printed in Great Britain by St Edmundsbury Press, Bury St Edmunds, Suffolk

ISBN 0 412 58110 8   1 56593 339 7 (USA)

A catalogue record for this book is available from the British Library

Library of Congress Catalog Card Number: 95–67598

∞ Printed on permanent acid-free text paper, manufactured in accordance with ANSI/NISO Z39.48-1992 and ANSI/NISO Z39.48-1984 (Permanence of Paper).

Contents

Contents   vii

Preface

As someone who was trained in the clinical scientific tradition it took me
several years to start to appreciate that food was more than a collection of
nutrients, and that most people did not make their choices of what to eat
on the biologically rational basis of nutritional composition. This realization helped to bring me to an understanding of why people didn't always
eat what (I believed) was good for them, and why the patients I had seen
in hospital as often as not had failed to follow the dietary advice I had so
confidently given.

When I entered the field of health education I quickly discovered the
famous World Health Organization definition of health as being a state of
complete physical, mental and social well-being, and not merely the
absence of disease. Health was a triangle – and I had been guilty of virtually ignoring two sides of that triangle. As I became involved in practical
nutrition education initiatives the deficiencies of an approach based on
giving information about nutrition and physical health became more and
more apparent. The children whom I saw in schools knew exactly what to
say when asked to describe a nutritious diet: they could recite the food
guide and list rich sources of vitamins and minerals; but none of this
intellectual knowledge was reflected in their own actual eating habits. Yet
nutrition education continued to focus on rote learning of nutrition information and food values. The situation in higher education did not seem
to be much different. The curriculum focused on physiological and
biochemical aspects of nutrition, while acknowledging only peripherally –
if at all – the non-biological meanings of food. This, I think, was a result of
a pervading medical model of nutrition which was disease prevention-
rather than health promotion-oriented. Within this context it should not
perhaps have been surprising that courses in sociology and psychology
were seen by many students as being largely irrelevant.

When I went to teach in Canada, a country where multiculturalism
flourishes, the importance of comprehending social meanings of food and
food-related behaviours was driven home even more forceably. In Britain
there had been some recent interest in developing nutrition education
materials suitable for use with Asian groups – a recognition of the obvious
cultural differences which existed in food patterns and preferences. In

Canada I had, in one class, students whose parents came from Germany, the Ukraine, Iceland, Malaya, Nigeria, Scotland, Norway, the USA ... the list seemed endless. Although the majority of these students were 'Canadians' they had grown up with quite different ideas of what constituted normal eating habits, what foods were acceptable on what occasions, what foods represented security, love, hospitality ... and so on. I was fortunate to be able to teach a course which dealt solely with the diversity of ethnic food habits and the cultural basis of food choice. It was from that experience that the idea for this book emerged, in which I have tried to cover a broad range of topics in sufficient detail to provide a basic appreciation of the non-biological reasons for food choice. If, as nutritionists, we gain only a small understanding of the role of food in society, we may be better able to put into perspective our own concerns for the metabolic adequacy of diets.

Human beings the world over share a common need to meet certain fundamental conditions for survival. One of these needs is the securing of an adequate diet which will provide energy and the various nutrients necessary for metabolic functioning. While the fact of this commonality may be so obvious as to hardly merit comment, it gives rise to an equally true but less readily appreciated observation. The range of human nutritional requirements is fairly narrow, but the ways in which these similar requirements are met are hugely diverse. Vastly differing dietary patterns, utilising thousands of different foodstuffs and combinations of foodstuffs are capable of achieving the same end – that of survival. It is also apparent that the body is able to call upon certain compensatory mechanisms to ensure short-term survival when nutritional needs are not being met. Biological adaptations have been described which act to conserve precious energy and body nutrient stores during periods of fasting or starvation; similarly, metabolic adjustments help to ensure successful outcome to pregnancy even where the mother is not optimally nourished. These are biological mechanisms; there are also culturally learnt adaptations designed to enhance survival prospects under adverse circumstances. Techniques of delaying or displacing hunger, for example, are important in societies where food shortages are common occurences.

The variety of substances which are consumed as food by various peoples of the world is truly remarkable; though for any given cultural group the list of acceptable foodstuffs is usually severely curtailed. The traditional Inuit diet consisted almost entirely of meat and fish; in many developing countries today, a single type of grain forms the bulk of what is eaten every day. In contrast, some North American Indian tribes traditionally ate over a hundred kinds of seeds, roots and nuts. In Europe and North America, meat comes mostly from beef, pork, lamb and chicken; but for the Dusan of Northern Borneo snake, gibbon, anteater, mouse and rat, are all acceptable protein sources. South American Indians eat monkeys, iguanas, grubs, bees and head lice, while the Aborigines of

Australasia relish insects. Fluids too come in a variety of forms: water, fruit juices, milk and blood; tea, coffee, cocoa, beer and wine. Non-food substances are regularly consumed; clay-eating practices among Mississippi Blacks: rotted wood consumption by the Vedda of Sri Lanka: pebble eating by the Guiana of South America - are examples. Sometimes humans learn to consume and to prefer substances which are intrinsically unpalatable. Coffee and chilli are flavours which have become widely desired despite the bitter and burning sensations they evoke. Rotted food is appreciated by the Dusan of Northern Borneo, who allow meat to spoil to liquefaction before consuming it with rice. The Vietnamese create sauces from putrified materials; sophisticated Europeans hang game birds until they are 'ripe'.

While the task of delineating 'what is eaten' is a far from simple one it is as nothing compared with addressing the question of 'why is it eaten?'. Food has always been much more than a source of body nourishment; it has played a major part in the social life, both religious and secular, of human groups. This book is intended to be a modest window into the world of food and culture. In gathering material and ideas, I was faced with an enormous range of potential topics and a bewilderingly array of sources from a wide cross-section of academic disciplines and popular publications. The selections I have made are therefore necessarily personal and somewhat arbitrary, though I have tried to illustrate what I see as major themes.

The second edition attempts to do three things:

- Elaborate and refine some of the material in the first edition, as a result of further reflections and in the light of more recent research and new information.
- Add new material and expand or re-organize existing material. Religion has been accorded a chapter of its own. There is a new chapter on 'Mass feeding' which examines aspects of food and popular culture, with special features on Japanese railway food, and the sub-culture of airline food. There is also a new chapter on gender issues and food. Elsewhere, new material is introduced on a variety of topics including: the legacy of the Columbian food exchange; the place of wild foods in the diet; festivals; and recipe repertoires.
- Be more accessible and useful to students and teachers, through a new format which includes special features, discussion questions, reading guides and illustrations.

A note to nutrition educators

Since the publication of the first edition of this book there have been a number of landmark events in the field of health and health promotion, charting the way to a 'new public health'. The Ottawa Charter for Health

Promotion in 1986 set out the fundamental principles and practice of health promotion, encompassing a much larger view of health than the medical focus on disease and health services with which we have become familiar. The World Health Organization's *Health for All by the Year 2000* and Canada's *Achieving Health for All* provided frameworks and mechanisms for action within this new vision.

> Health is the extent to which an individual or group can, on the one hand meet needs and realize aspirations and, on the other hand cope with the environment. It is a resource for every day living.

The concept of health is thus changing from absence of disease to the notion of control over one's own decisions and one's destiny. This changing paradigm has and will continue to affect the practice of nutrition which, as it becomes more oriented to health promotion principles, will focus more on supporting people in making their own healthy food choices and less on attempting to command obedience to professional prescriptions. To succeed in this endeavour, nutrition practitioners will have a greater need for a better understanding of the biocultural nature of eating. Already, calls for cultural sensitivity are becoming commonplace in the endless streams of reports and recommendations which flow from a multitude of task forces, working groups and expert advisory bodies. However, cultural sensitivity in nutrition must go beyond issues of literacy and language and inclusion of 'ethnic' foods in nutriton education materials. It must accomodate other ways of seeing the world. Food habits are not to be studied and understood simply so they can be changed. Rather, through developing an appreciation of the role that food plays in peoples lives, nutrition educators may become both more relevant and more effective.

For the reader who is neither nutritionist nor student, but who picks up the book through a general interest in food and people, my hope is that they will enjoy the feast. The multi-course menu of potlatches, hunger strikes, festivals, sacrifices, taboos, and dinner parties, should provide sustenance enough, but if attention wanes, then remember – there's always the coffee pot and the biscuit tin....

Winnipeg, 1994

Acknowledgements

I am indebted to my Japanese colleague and translator, Dr Kohmei Wani for his comments on material in the book and for his invaluable assistance in providing background material and photographs for the Ekiben section of Chapter 10. I am grateful to the airline representatives who responded to my request for information on food service and who provided sample menus and other materials. Dr John Guilfoyle provided the impetus for and advised on the presentation of the Ba'hai section of Chapter 6. I was constantly encouraged by the editorial staff at Chapman & Hall and I would particularly like to acknowledge Lisa Fraley and Catherine Walker for their support and advice.

Finally, I owe a great thank you to my wife, Corinne Eisenbraun, who not only read critically every version of the evolving manuscript, but also made it possible for me to devote the time necessary to complete the writing. My thanks also to Emma and Veronica, who patiently accepted the news that 'Daddy's in the basement again'.

Responsibility for errors and omissions are mine alone, and I remain conscious of the debt owed to the many authors on whose work I have drawn in this volume.

Biocultural perspectives on nutrition

In no area of biology is the relationship with the social sciences more inclusive or critical than in the nutritional sciences.

RICHARD BARNES *(1968)*

FOOD AND CULTURE

Even a cursory glance through the scientific and humanities literature, or a modicum of reflective thought is enough to produce ready agreement with the idea that culture is a major determinant of what we eat. Whereas it is easily seen that the direct consequences of food intake are biological – food meets the energy and nutrient needs of the body – it is also apparent that the nature of that food intake is shaped by a wide variety of geographical, social, psychological, religious, economic and political factors. Recognition of the fact that food intake is a response to both biological and cultural stimuli and that eating fulfils both biological and social needs leads inescapably to the conclusion that the study of nutrition is a biocultural issue par excellence. Foods chosen, methods of eating, preparation, number of meals per day, time of eating and the size of portions eaten make up human foodways and are an integrated part of a coherent cultural pattern in which each custom and practice has a part to play. Food habits come into being and are maintained because they are practical or symbolically meaningful behaviours in a particular culture although this may not be readily apparent to the casual observer. They are a product of ecological forces acting within the context of historical conditioning and belief systems – a melding of new ideas and imperatives with old traditions.

When we use the term culture in everyday speech we often employ it as a convenient shorthand for an ill-defined entity which we might better describe as way of life. We are vaguely aware that our culture is what makes us similar to some other people and yet different from the vast majority of people in the world. It is a kind of social heritage. Moreover, we usually distinguish this usage of the word from the artistic vision of culture and from the notion of culture as that which is refined, sophisticated and highbrow. It nevertheless defies precise definition. Anthropologists too, have disagreed about the meaning of culture. Although many different attempts at formulations have been made over the years, Tylor's early definition is still useful; culture is that complex whole which includes knowledge, belief, art, morals, law, customs, and any other capabilities and habits acquired by man as a member of society (Tylor, 1871). And indeed it is complex, being the sum total of a group's learned, shared behaviour. The terms culture and society are sometimes used interchangeably; whereas it is true that there can be no culture apart from society they are nevertheless not the same thing. Culture describes patterns of behaviour; society refers to the people who participate in the culture and thus give it concrete expression.

Although there is great diversity between cultures, a number of characteristics applicable to all cultures may be identified (Foster, 1962). Culture is a learned experience; it is acquired by people as they live their everyday lives. It is not biologically determined and therefore can be modified or unlearned. Culture is a group phenomenon, not an individual one; it is transmitted from one generation to the next and in the absence of socialization processes would not be continued. It may be transmitted formally or informally by verbal instruction or by non-verbal cues and through personal example.

Culture involves change; each generation, although it learns the culture it is born into, is never exactly the same as its predecessor. Culture is not static; it preserves traditions but also builds in mechanisms for change. Food habits are part of this dynamic process in that whereas they are basically stable and predictable they are, paradoxically, at the same time undergoing constant and continuous change. Change occurs over time because of ecological and economic changes leading to altered availability, discovery or innovation of foods and diffusion or borrowing of food habits from others. Rao (1986) coins the term **gastrodynamics** to refer to such changing dietary styles and food behaviour. Notwithstanding this, every culture resists change; food habits, though far from fixed, are also far from easy to change.

We are, on the whole, unconscious of our culture. It is internalized so that most of our routine behaviours are done unthinkingly, simply because that's how they are done. We may even be unaware that there are rules governing many aspects of our behaviour. We internalize cultural traditions so that they become an inseparable part of our self-identity, and few of us realize to what extent we are creatures of the cultural traditions in which we were raised.

Culture has a value system. Dominant values will influence all aspects of food-related activity as well as the way specific foods are viewed. Among the substances accepted as food by a culture some are labelled good and some bad. Bad foods are sometimes highly desired, as in the case of empty calorie so-called 'junk foods'.

In addition to the above universals, a culture contains symbols that are understood by the group, which emphasize specific activities, and which provide for interaction between people in a socially acceptable manner. If there is a widespread failure of culturally sanctioned behaviour patterns to meet the needs of people, then the cultural norms which dictate acceptable behaviour may be overthrown. Food riots and antisocial behaviour during food shortages are consequences of the inadequacy of established social and economic mechanisms in dealing with abnormal situations. For example, in late 18th century Burgundy bread riots occurred in response to price rises and as part of a growing anti-seigneural protest over who controlled the produce of the land. During the revolution the hungry crowd became a vehicle for forcing constitutional change although, in the end, the revolution did not actually resolve the problems of feeding 28 million French people (Rotberg, 1983). Cultural norms may also be over-ridden when necessity dictates. Cannibalism is looked upon with revulsion by most societies but is tolerated when circumstances make it the only hope of survival.

Urbanization, the rise of agribusiness and the growing impact of international trade in foodstuffs have undermined the ability of people to practise self-sufficiency in meeting their food needs. The complex cash-based food system of modern industrialized nations removes most people from a direct role in food production and puts them at the mercy of an intricate food distribution network. There is a danger that this system cannot meet the food needs of all segments of the population as evidenced by increasing numbers of reports of malnutrition in affluent communities and the appearance of food banks and other forms of food relief in ostensibly rich northern cities. If abnormal situations become common enough, there will be pressure for changes in cultural patterns to accommodate the new reality. Perhaps people will maintain food security by rediscovering the merits of regional and local food systems and becoming more self-reliant again.

In the next section the universal attributes of culture identified above are further discussed specifically as they apply to food habits.

Socialization and acquisition of food habits

Culture is learned. Food habits are acquired early in life and once established are likely to be long-lasting and resistant to change. Hence the importance of developing sound nutritional practices in childhood as a basis for life-long healthy eating. Socialization describes the process by which culturally valued norms of behaviour are passed on from generation to generation. It is a life-long process; natural functions such as eating become socialized as the growing child is conditioned by customs and traditions. Some authors distinguish between socialization – the transmission of culture, and enculturation – transmission of a specific culture. The early acquisition of food habits and the implications of this process for nutrition education has been discussed elsewhere (Fieldhouse, 1983). Of equal importance to the learning of what we may call nutritional values is the concurrent learning of social values attached to food and food events. Table 1.1 depicts the socialization process as applied to food habits.

Table 1.1 Socialization and the acquisition of food habits

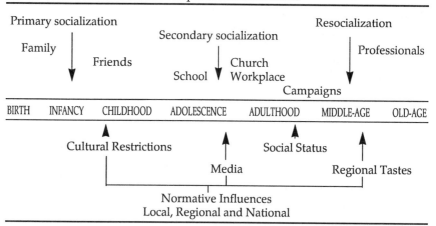

*Resocialization refers to change and is thus more of a consideration in adult life as indicated in the diagram. It can however apply at any time throughout the life span. Similarly, normative influences are always present though they may be more or less powerful at different times of life.

Primary socialization occurs mainly through the agency of the immediate family. The infant and young child are dependent on adults for what they get to eat and food is one of the basic mediums through which adult attitudes and sentiments are communicated. Children have to learn to like what is prescribed by the culinary culture in which they are raised; they have little choice in the matter other than through the refusal to eat at all. Appropriate or desired behaviour is reinforced whereas deviant or undesired behaviour is sanctioned. Young children have a preference for foods which are sweet and which are familiar. Although it seems reasonable to suppose that parental example is important in getting children to accept unfamiliar foods, resemblance in parent–child preferences is quite low. This gives rise to a paradox; if the child develops food preferences through cultural learning then why are the parents not more influential? If most of the intra-cultural variance in individual food preferences is influenced by the environment other than the family, then what is its source? (Rozin, 1990). One explanation may lie with the pervasive influence of mass media (see below). Early eating experiences readily become associated with family sentiments, of happiness and warmth or of anger and tension; it is not surprising then that foods acquire the power to unlock childhood memories when they are encountered in later life.

As children grow older they are exposed to diverse experiences and viewpoints and to multiple influences. Socializing agencies may complement or conflict with one another. For example, food habits which have been informally learnt at home are either reinforced or contradicted in the more formal setting of the school. The law of primacy implies that those habits learnt earliest are most likely to persist in later life and to be most resistant to change; thus when there is a conflict, say between what is taught at school and what is taught in the home, the latter is most likely to dominate. This reinforces the idea that the creation of early likes and dislikes congruent with healthy eating habits is a desirable nutrition strategy.

Resocialization is an attempt to usurp old routines and practices and replace them with new ones. Typically it occurs through educational and intervention programmes designed by health professionals. Eating habits may change if sufficient benefit is demonstrated, though the failure rate of such change attempts is notoriously high. In the light of this more attention is now being given to a variety of different change strategies ranging from community development to healthy public policy.

Depicted in the lower part of Table 1.1 are various normative influences operating throughout the lifespan. These factors affect all members of the society to a greater or lesser extent. Thus cultural restrictions define for everyone what constitutes food; for example, children in Britain or Canada quickly learn that earthworms are not regarded as being edible. Regional tastes result in selective exposure to foods which in turn shape preferences and subsequent food choice patterns. Advertising of food products may have a considerable impact on food requests by children and on purchasing behaviour by adults. Indeed, in industrialized countries food marketing strategies may be more powerful than rational experience or traditional practices in influencing food habits (Abrahamsson, 1979).

In addition to imparting food values the socialization process teaches social, cultural and psychological meanings and uses of food. Table 1.2 depicts a paradigm for socialization of food meanings. Children are not mere recipients of a complex code of food regulations passed down through socializing agencies; they are often the agency through which new food practices or products are introduced to a family or social group. Practices learnt in school may be carried back into the home. Because children are usually permitted a greater degree of latitude in deviancy from accepted habits, new or strange food practices are more readily tolerated and may eventually become accepted and incorporated into mainstream food behaviour.

Biocultural perspectives on nutrition

Table 1.2 Socialization and food usages

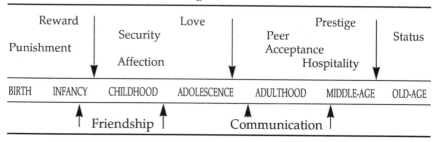

| Reward Punishment | Security Affection | Love | Peer Acceptance | Prestige Hospitality | Status |

| BIRTH | INFANCY | CHILDHOOD | ADOLESCENCE | ADULTHOOD | MIDDLE-AGE | OLD-AGE |

Friendship   Communication

While the learning of various social meanings of food is a continuous process, particular values or usages may be emphasized at different stages of the life span. The role of food in friendship and communication may be considered to be a 'normative' meaning, operating most of the time.

Change

It is true that while food habits are often inculcated early in life and are on the whole stable and long-lasting they are nevertheless subject to change, perhaps as a consequence of changing physical or social environments or perhaps as a result of educational programmes or medical intervention. Some examples are given below, beginning with the phenomenon known as acculturation.

Acculturation

Acculturation refers to the process by which groups and individuals adapt to the norms and values of an alien culture. It is induced by contact with foreign cultures and the process is usually two-way with, however, one culture dominating. For example, migrants generally tend to adopt the food habits prevalent in the place of destination, though this is mediated in many ways (Rao, 1986). They may recreate their own culinary culture in the new homeland, making compromises and substitutions for ingredients no longer available. They may also bring essential foods and equipment from their place of origin. They may become bipalatal, choosing to eat local foods in public while retaining their own cuisine at home. Not only the actual foods consumed change but there are accompanying changes in beliefs, attitudes and social uses of foods. The degree of change experienced is related to the social context of migration including living conditions, new social networks and the strength of ties maintained with the place of origin. Food habits change most rapidly among the young who are subject to school and work peer influences, and where there is little cultural support for the old ways. Thus an East Indian family settling into a British industrial city such as Birmingham or Bradford, where there is already a stable ethnic community, might be expected to retain traditional practices much longer than Vietnamese Boat-People who find themselves relocated in rural Saskatchewan, or young single students adjusting to the multiple demands of an overseas university education.

Rao (1986) presents case studies of five streams of migrants in India. One of these concerns Malayalee migrants from Kerala to Delhi who are faced with a shift from a culinary culture based on rice, fish, tapioca, banana and coconut oil to one where wheat is staple, fish and coconut are rare and mustard oil is used for cooking. The presence of the new migrants created a demand for a factory-produced neutral tasting vegetable cooking oil to replace scarce coconut oil. Over time previously central foods became peripheral and cooking practices changed as certain special cooking vessels were hard to get. Even meal etiquette changed from squatting to the use of a dining table. However, traditional food habits were retained for ritual occasions such as feasts, fasts and large communal meals.

The impact of acculturation on food habits over several generations is well illustrated in a comparison of ethnic Swiss living in Switzerland and Brazil (Uhle and Grivetti, 1993). An immigrant group from Obwalden, Switzerland, escaping the potato famines of Europe, founded Colonia Helvetia in Brazil in the 1850s. A contemporary study of food habits in the two populations showed varying levels of cultural change in foodways, as indicated by the names and ingredients used for dishes. The Brazilian–Swiss population still retained some German speciality items in both name and substance, for example Apfelmues, or applesauce; in other cases either the name or the ingredients, or both, of the original German dish had become transformed into Portuguese substitutes while some traditional 19th century German dishes had disappeared altogether and indigenous Portuguese dishes had been adopted. The study, as the authors point out, demonstrates how food contributes to creating ethnic unity in culturally isolated population groups, to the extent that common ethnic food practices can still be seen after a century of geographic and cultural removal from the homeland.

There are numerous examples of acculturation processes which have produced negative nutritional effects. Inuit villagers, exposed to White North American culture consequent on oil-field exploration in the Arctic, have suffered an erosion of their traditional lifestyles. From being a basically hunting and gathering culture they have become more and more dependent on prepared foods sold in stores. This process began when fur-traders began to infiltrate remote areas and when trading posts were established. Game became less available, and hunting was made easier with the introduction of firearms. As permanent White communities grew up, native peoples were more and more influenced by the cultural values of the outsiders. Eating the White Man's food was a source of prestige. Today we see extensive examples of malnutrition where traditional food habits have been abandoned in favour of a limited diet of largely empty-calorie foods. A good example of the effects of the acculturation process is provided by contrasting descriptions of two Inuit communities, one exposed to urban values and the other retaining a more traditional lifestyle (Schaefer *et al.*, 1980). A comparison of Arctic Bay, a small eastern Arctic settlement following largely traditional practices, with Inuvik, an urbanized western Arctic centre established during the oil boom of the 1950s, revealed a pattern of ill-health in Inuvik native peoples similar to that seen in industrialized North America and which was not prevalent in the more isolated community of Arctic Bay.

Another example is furnished by the Dene (Chipewyan) Indians of Northern Canada, who were traditionally a hunting and fishing society. With the development of the fur-trading economy, fishing and hunting became intensified and food resources were consequently depleted. As the Dene settled in permanent communities they developed increasing reliance on staples of the White traders, bought at the local store (Schaefer and Steckle, 1980). In discussing the impact of socioeconomic changes on the traditional diets of Cree Indians from Eastern James Bay, Berkes and Farkas (1978) recommended a rejuvenation of traditional food habits as well as an increase in the quality of store-bought food in order to preserve adequate standards of nutrition. Since then the situation in remote northern communities has, if anything, worsened and similar calls are being made today.

In a different time and place, an example of acculturation leaving a permanent mark on food usages is seen in the language of food itself. The English names of ox, cow, calf, pig, sheep, boar and deer are used to describe living animals; when these animals are cooked and served at table they bear the French names of beef, veal, pork, bacon, mutton, brawn and venison. This difference is often attributed to the fact that in Medieval times the lower classes were responsible for keeping the animals, whereas the upper classes did most of the actual meat eating. The influence of the Norman conquest in England resulted in adoption of French manners and customs, particularly among the aristocratic classes and hence the use of French food names at the table. Vestiges of this manifestation of social distinction may be seen in modern up-market restaurants, where the menu is ostentatiously written or printed in French.

Changing cultural patterns

Dietary changes do not necessarily have to be externally induced. Shifts in cultural patterns and values within a society inevitably affect or are reflected in dietary practices. One of the most profound of these in industrialized countries is a continuing change in family structures and working arrangements. The traditional extended family system is rapidly disappearing, and with it the concept of set meal times to be eaten in the company of specified family members. The nuclear family consisting of mother, father and children is a more flexible, mobile unit in which eating can be and is an individual non-scheduled event (Sanjur, 1982). The nuclear family itself represents a diminishing proportion of households as one-parent families and live-in arrangements become more common. When single parents and married women take employment outside the home, whether by choice or through economic necessity, other family members become more responsible for their own diets. Eating out has also become more economically feasible and is suited to modern hectic lifestyles. In Canada about 40 cents of every dollar is spent on food eaten out of the home.

While the family structure has contracted and fragmented, the food supply has expanded dramatically. The phenomenon of delocalization describes a trend away from self-sufficiency and community to mass production and globalization. In comparing the food system of a modern industrialized country to that of 50 years ago, Kuhnlein (1992) comments that there is a greater range of raw foods; a greater diversity of prepared (processed) foods; less use of local products; greater homogenization within regions of a country and mass standardization of agricultural products. In contrast to these, and perhaps in reaction to them there is also a revived interest in ethnic cuisine. The number of new food products introduced in Canada doubled in the 5 years from 1986–1991, and the Canadian shopper now has over 11 000 products to choose from in a conventional supermarket and maybe 17 000 in a superstore. It is not surprising therefore that pre-prepared convenience foods form a large and growing part of the average diet. In critiquing this illusion of choice in relation to women's roles as food providers, Gussow (1986) notes that people (mostly women) spend endless unnecessary hours in supermarkets making pointless discriminations between basically identical products.

Many would agree with Gussow that the complex global food system does not serve to ensure that the majority of people are adequately nourished – a failure which, moreover, is accompanied by a profligate waste of resources. Arable land is removed from the control of peasant farmers growing subsistence crops and diverted to producing luxury cash crops for rich consumers in faraway countries; incredible human effort and ingenuity is combined with huge inputs of raw materials and energy to fuel a food industry which provides a surfeit of nutritionally useless products; fresh fruits and vegetables are discarded by the tonne and left to rot if they don't meet the quality standards of wholesale purchasers. As concern for the integrity of the environment becomes a public issue, conservation of food and energy resources gains increasing attention among those who give thought to the meaning of food security. Many people have given expression to these concerns by deliberately reducing their consumption of material goods and services, rejecting consumerist values and adopting simpler lifestyles. This has spurred an increased interest in local food security strategies, such as family and community gardens, food co-operatives and shared farming, which recapture a modicum of community control over food supply.

Continuing preoccupation with health and physical fitness gives rise to weight consciousness, ever-changing fad diets, and planned calorie-controlled regimes by the thousand. North Americans and Europeans are continually bombarded with messages exhorting them to seek ultimate fitness. Part and parcel of this quest is the search for health foods – whether they come from organic gardens or the shelves of health stores which thrive on massive sales of diet supplements and pills. Recently, more attention has been given both to the lack of efficacy of most slimming diets and their potential for actually creating health risks. Now that there are signs of a shift of attitude among health professionals regarding the wisdom and value of dieting it remains to be seen whether changes in public attitudes and practices follow.

Despite trends toward greater homogeneity of food supply there are also signs of increasing interest in and acceptance of ethnic foods. Whereas the United States has opted for a **melting pot** policy, and Canada has stressed the **cultural mosaic** approach, in both countries there is a tremendous mix of ethnic and cultural groups each with its own particular foodways. Acculturation of minorities, accompanied by an increased interest in cultural heritage and self-identity has promoted the popularity of ethnic foods, some of which have become American staples. The shopping malls of North America are enlivened with an endless selection of cafes and fast-food outlets selling such favourites as tacos, pyroghies, chow mein, patties and pizzas as well as the ubiquitous burger. Here is a good example of the two-way nature of acculturation.

A major facet of social change in the last few decades has been in the communications industry. In a comparatively short time, members of industrialized societies have progressed from being dependent on occasional printed material and oral reporting as sources of information to a point where they have instantaneous access to news of worldwide events distributed by a complex and technologically sophisticated communications system. The imminent arrival of computerized electronic highways promises (or threatens) an almost unlimited capacity for communication and information dissemination. Currently, the channels through which this rapid communication is effected are collectively known as the mass media. Television, radio, newspapers and magazines are the main channels, with television being predominant. The ubiquity of the television set in the homes of industrialized nations and increasingly in towns and villages of developing countries has turned it into a powerful means of disseminating information. The potential for television as a medium for health promotion was acknowledged in a recent US Government report (US Department of Health and Human Services, 1991), while in Canada several proposals have been developed for 24-hour health channels. Canadian researchers recently claimed that television has three sorts of impact on nutrition. Firstly, through feature programming and advertising, it provides information and possibly educates the audience. Secondly, it contributes to the establishment of social norms for body image. Thirdly, through its passive nature it encourages a sedentary lifestyle; the average Canadian watches over 20 hours of television a week (Østbye et al., 1993). Not surprisingly, those with something to sell have identified television advertising as a potent tool.

Mass media, advertising and food habits

The role of the media in shaping food habits is a controversial one. As an impersonal communication channel is more effective in conveying information than in active persuasion some would claim that mass media impact is limited simply to making people aware of what is available. This view would suggest that a television advertisement only affects those who are already predisposed to buy the product and does not induce a desire for previously unwanted items. Advertising may indeed influence choice of brand-name or specific commodity within an already desired category of items. Thus if I intend to buy a car and see an advertisement for a recent model then I may be inclined to examine that model for possible purchase. Similarly, if I intend to purchase a cake mix or a can of soup, adverts may push particular brands to the forefront of my mind, so that when actual purchases are made these brands are likely to be selected. However, if I have no desire to eat canned soups, then no amount of advertising is going to persuade me to buy that product. This line of thought reflects the belief that mass media advertising can do no more than provide information – and that information alone is an insufficient motivation for action. The latter is certainly true; but there are those who would maintain that advertising does do more than provide information.

Certainly advertisers are prepared to make huge financial investments in short television commercials, believing that this technique does indeed sell products. They expect that advertising will not only increase overall product consumption but will also specifically increase their market share by establishing product identity and building brand loyalty. The audience for such advertisements is extremely large. Hanssen (1980) said of advertising that it 'persuades us that the right taste for a food is the result of some particular concept designed by marketing men, created by food technologists and produced in beautiful factories, with sales potential as the guiding light, rather than nutritional consequences.' In a similar vein, C.W. Post, founder of General Foods was reported as saying 'You can't just manufacture cereal. You've got to get it halfway down the customer's throat through advertising. Then they've got to swallow it.' (Peoples Food Commission, 1980).

Advocates of food advertising claim that it stimulates competition and keeps prices down; opponents maintain that the huge sums spent on advertising inevitably increase the price of a product. Nutritional concerns are raised because many of the products most heavily advertised are low in nutritional value. The commercial promotion of food products does not, on the whole, focus on the nutritional value of a product or the contribution it makes to physiological well-being. Rather advertising utilizes powerful symbolic meanings of foods, so that what is being sold is not just a product, but a lifestyle, a dream, a source of emotional fulfilment (Table 1.3).

Table 1.3 Marketing appeals in food advertising

The food itself:	Convenience
	Newness
	Naturalness
	Traditional
	Nutritional value
Economics:	Cost
	Value for money
	'Specials'
	Economy packs
Food as a means to something else:	Status value
	Endorsement by celebrities
	Popularity
	Ideal mother/wife
	Sexual attraction
	Fitness and slimness
	Reward
	Success

Analysis of advertisements on five Canadian TV channels, public and private, English and French, local and national revealed that commercials for foods and food products constituted one-quarter to one-third of all ads, making them the single largest sector of products advertised. The most common ads were for beer and wine, followed by complete meals such as pasta and sauce, frozen dinners, hamburgers, pizza and soups. The predominant grain product advertised was breakfast cereals; there were no ads for fresh vegetables and only one for fruit (apples). Much Music, a music video channel aimed at teenagers and young adults, was dominated by ads for soft drinks, sweets and alcohol (Østbye *et al.*, 1993).

Of particular concern is the role of mass media advertising in the formation of children's foods habits. Many advertisements are specifically targeted at children and feature confectionery, soft drinks and snack foods. The Canadian study mentioned above found that on the national private network during Saturday morning children's programmes a half of all advertisements were for foods and food products. Breakfast cereals, french fries, fish sticks, canned spaghetti and ketchup topped the list, with fast food restaurants close behind. Advertisers hope to persuade the child to put pressure on parents to buy brand-name products. Young children may not be able to distinguish between adverts and programmes, and certainly do not have the sophistication to decry fact from fiction. Older children can, especially if guided, recognize the essentially unreal nature of adverts. The amount of research in this area is limited, possibly by the difficulties inherent in assessing the diffuse impact of mass media channels. However it is evident that children are exposed to a large amount of food advertising, that the products advertised are mostly low nutrient foods, and that this does have an impact on children's food preferences and behaviours.

Resistance to change

Although change is inevitable, and is indeed essential to the well-being of a society, it is true that resistance to change is often widespread and difficult to overcome. The introduction of a new idea or practice may be termed an innovation and it usually originates from an external source. Whether the innovation is accepted or not, and the speed at which it diffuses throughout a society is dependent on a variety of factors associated both with the nature of the innovation and the nature of the society into which it is introduced. Five characteristics of innovations may be identified and briefly discussed in relation to food habits; these are, relative advantage, compatibility, complexity, trialability and observability.

- The greater the perceived relative advantage of an innovation, the more rapid its rate of adoption. Obviously a proposed change must be seen to have more advantages than drawbacks, unless it is to be enforced rather than being a matter of voluntary adoption.
- Compatibility is the degree to which an innovation is perceived as being consistent with the existing values and needs of society members. In the field of nutritional health many examples of incompatibility could be cited. For example; the promotion of beef as a good protein source in school classes of Hindu children; the advocacy of margarine as a source of vitamin D for Indian immigrants; the promotion of citrus fruit to the elderly – many of whom believe these foods are 'acid' and will harm them. The adoption of an incompatible innovation requires the prior adoption of a new belief or value system.
- Complexity is the degree to which an innovation is perceived as being difficult to understand and use. Those innovations which require little effort from the recipient will be adopted more rapidly than those demanding new skills and understanding. Where little effort is combined with much gain ready adoption may be expected, as in the case of an ulcer patient directed to forego fried foods.

- Trialability is the degree to which an innovation may be experimented with on a limited basis. A trialable innovation represents less risk to the individual or group which is considering it. Substituting artificial sweetener for sugar is eminently trialable, whereas fluoridation is not.
- Observability is the degree to which the results of an innovation are visible to others. The easier it is for individuals to see the results of an innovation, the more likely they are to adopt it permanently. Many desirable health behaviours do not have observable effects because they are, in essence, preventive actions. Thus it is very difficult to demonstrate, at an individual level, the potential benefits of a particular dietary pattern in preventing coronary heart disease or gastrointestinal disorders.

The rate of adoption of an innovation by a social group is usually measured by the length of time required for a certain percentage of the group to adopt the innovation. Members of the group are often classified as innovators, early adopters, early majority, late majority and laggards. Social systems typified by modern, rather than traditional norms exhibit faster rates of adoption. According to Rogers and Shoemaker (1971), a social system with modern norms is more change-oriented, technologically developed, scientific, rational, cosmopolite and empathic. This suggests that not only will food innovations be more readily accepted in industrialized countries, but also that they will have most impact among the higher socioeconomic groups of a society. In both Britain and North America for example, it has been well recognized that the modern trend toward breastfeeding is most marked among women from social classes I and II – the same groups who led the move to bottle feeding 40 years ago.

Unintended impact of food innovations on society

Just as social trends can influence food habits, so when changes in food usages occur there may result widespread and unexpected changes in other, non-food related aspects of society.

Many attempts to increase agricultural production, under the banner of development, rely on increased labour inputs. For example, HYV crops (High-Yielding Varieties) introduced during the Green Revolution made extra demands on women for planting, transplanting seedlings and especially for weeding. Additional tasks such as hoeing and ridging were sometimes necessary. At the same time as such planned innovations in agriculture impose extra work on women they reduce demands on men through mechanization of land clearance, ploughing and harvesting. Rogers (1981) cites evidence that the simultaneous reduction of men's labour and increase of women's labour leads to increased hostility between men and women and raises general tensions within the family.

Innovations may also adversely affect the nutritional value of the diet. The introduction of wheat and potatoes into the Bangladeshi rice agricultural cycle displaced cultivation of many varieties of pulse and millet. Thus while wheat contains more protein than rice, the decline in pulse consumption it triggered meant a net shift to protein of inferior quality (Lindenbaum 1986).

Our unconscious culture

As a result of socialization processes many of our everyday decisions become routinized; that is they are performed as a matter of habit, without conscious deliberation. We understand that cereals are proper breakfast foods and that milk is good to drink without having to be reminded every day. More fundamentally, we know what is and what is not food; we may deliberate over a choice between carrots and cauliflower, but not between chicken and snake. Some nutrition educators argue that the creation of sound nutrition routines, which are internalized during the period of primary socialization, holds out the greatest promise of success for long term nutritional health.

Values

The value system of a culture shapes the way in which foods are used. A total culture is composed of many parts or subsystems, each of which has an impact on individual food behaviour. Sometimes the interaction of subsystems may give rise to conflicting values. Bass *et al.* (1979) identify subsystems in North America as being ideological; technological; economic; educational; political; family; mass media. Some of the value implications these have for food behaviour are listed in Table 1.4. Minority groups, whether they be defined in social, cultural or ethnic terms may hold values which differ from those of the dominant culture and this is reflected in their beliefs, attitudes and practices related to food.

Success in designing programmes to influence food patterns is enhanced by the realization that nutritional practices are largely determined by basic customs which are, in turn, inter-related with other aspects of social organization. For example, Freedman (1977) cites studies of the Polela Zulus of Natal, where initial efforts to promote use of eggs and milk among the Polela were resisted due to complex kinship rules and practical economics. Subsequently, beliefs regarding eggs were identified: to eat an egg which would later hatch was uneconomical; eating eggs was a sign of greed; eating eggs made young girls lascivious. By taking measures to increase the productivity of the hens, the first of these barriers was overcome; further persuasion and education resulted in a weakening of the other, less important rationales, and eventually in the adoption of egg eating. In another example, from Chile, powdered milk

Table 1.4 Impact of cultural subsystems on food values

Ideological	Humans have the right to control the earth's resources to their own ends It is good to feed the poor and underprivileged
Technological	Humans can solve world food problems through the application of ever-more sophisticated technology Greater energy inputs are needed to produce food
Economic	Food is treated as a commodity with a specific monetary value Food supply and distribution occurs independently of actual human need
Education	Food knowledge, beliefs and attitudes are transmitted from on generation to the next Research efforts are directed to improving the food supply
Political	Government regulations affect production, trade, distribution, safety and quality of food
Family	Each family member directly influences the food habits of the others Changes in the diet of one family member has repercussions for the rest of the family
Mass media	Food habits are shaped by a powerful socialising agency Food products are promoted selectively on a non-nutritional basis

introduced at health clinics was provided free to needy families. It was initially rejected as it was suspected to be of poor quality or to be harmful, but a small charge made it quite acceptable. A similar phenomenon is sometimes seen in Britain, in health clinics which offer nutrition programmes and free dietary advice. The 'free' service is judged to be inferior to the programmes of commercial slimming organizations. Underlying this is the attitude that you get what you pay for (even though most people are at least aware that they have already indirectly paid for public services through their taxes). Many more examples in the nutritional and anthropological literature attest to the importance of understanding cultural values and norms if nutrition innovations are to be successfully introduced.

At the same time one should never underestimate human ingenuity. When the Italian government supplied a shipment of macaroni to Salvadorean refugees living in a Honduran refugee camp, there was neither the cultural context nor the appropriate cuisine accompaniments to prepare it 'Italian-style'. However, through experimentation the Salvadoreans discovered that macaroni deep-fried in fat produced an acceptable nutty snack. Toasted and pulverized it could be mixed with cinnamon, sugar and water to make a refreshing drink, while by first grinding it into flour, the pasta could be baked into bread (Schlabach, 1991).

FOOD HABIT RESEARCH

Having reviewed the cultural context of food habits the remainder of this chapter is devoted to an overview of methodological approaches to, and models of, human food selection.

Early American studies on food habits were carried out in the 1920s and 1930s, culminating in the formation of the US National Research Council Committee on Food Habits. Because of the impending threat of war the government was interested in how food habits could be changed if rationing became necessary to deal with possible food shortages. Kurt Lewin and Margaret Mead were prominent names in the early history of this committee whose work included the production of a handbook which was, in effect, a procedure manual for gathering data (Committee on Food Habits, 1945), and which still has relevance today. In the ensuing decades a number of different approaches to the study of food habits emerged.

Food habit researchers use a variety of approaches to gather information. The method employed reflects on the viewpoint of the researcher and colours the results or the interpretations drawn from results. Thus it is often difficult to compare findings of different studies and it is also easy to find conflicting interpretations of the same cultural phenomena. Grivetti and Pangborn (1973) have summarized the most popular methodologies, while Messer (1984) also provides a useful account of different anthropological approaches to diet. Two broad perspectives may be referred to as the materialist and the mentalist. Materialists attempt to define food habits in terms of biological or ecological imperatives, whereas mentalists are interested in the symbolic meanings and uses of food.

Materialist approaches which view food habits as being determined by the environment have been largely abandoned, as they treat humans as passive creatures taking whatever food is available. Numerous examples throughout this book will show that simple availability is not a good basis from which to predict food habits. Recognizing the shortcomings of the environmentalist stance, cultural ecologists have emphasized the dynamic interaction of humans with their environment. Physical and geographical conditions lead to certain types of food getting and agricultural systems, which in turn lead to models of social organization and rituals calculated to improve food production (Back, 1977). Thus culturally framed food habits serve to meet ecological, nutritional or economic ends. While cultural ecologists can explain the nutritional value of a particular cultural practice a statement of causality or origin cannot be derived from that explanation. Moreover, as ecology is concerned with human adaptation to an environment it is not clear what constitutes successful adaption, who in a society adapts, and at what cost (Kahn, 1986). Finally, cultural ecology tends to ignore or play down social and religious elements of food practices. Nevertheless, the approach has yielded valuable insights into food habits and some of the more attractive cultural ecology theories are discussed in detail in later chapters.

The culture–history approach is based on analysis of evidence from archaeological, linguistic, historical and oral tradition sources to trace the origins and spread of dietary practices. Most historical nutrition studies restrict themselves to a specific geographical area, a specific food or a specific time period.

Mentalist approaches employ symbolic analysis to relate food categorization and food-related behaviour to deeper structures of the mind. What people believe and do regarding food reveals how they think about the world. From a functionalist perspective, food is a vehicle for social communication. Food habits satisfy particular social needs and stabilize social relationships. Using this approach researchers have often been able to identify reasons for apparently irrational food-related behaviours and resistance to attempts to change existing food habits.

Probably no single approach provides all the information necessary for a full understanding of food habits. A fusion or combination of approaches, and collaboration between researchers working in multi-disciplinary teams would be of immense value. Cattle (1977) also condemns what she calls nutritional particularism. She says that it has hindered interdisciplinary cooperation, and has resulted in the generation of discrete and disconnected units of information. As an alternative to particularism she proposes an adaptive model which embraces biological, evolutionary, ecological and sociocultural processes. Many other authors also stress the need to integrate sociocultural and biologic approaches to the study of nutrition (see for example Pelto and Jerome, 1978).

Nutritional anthropology

Applied nutritional anthropology may be defined as the application of anthropological data and methods to the solving of the cultural aspects of human nutrition problems, or as the study of the interrelationships between diet and culture and their mutual influence upon one another (Freedman, 1977). Anthropologists have tended to view food practices simply as one element of the set of customs which makes up a culture, without necessarily being concerned about the impact of these practices on health. Nutritionists on the other hand have focused on the health effects and have not been greatly concerned with cultural values regarding food (Krondl and Boxen, 1975). Anthropological reports have traditionally been qualitative in nature; nutritionists have favoured quantitative approaches, describing the dietary habits and nutritional status of populations in statistical terms. A marriage of these two approaches promises fruitful research efforts within the emerging discipline known as nutritional anthropology. For example, Khare and Rao (1986) suggest that a comprehensive ethnography of food should concern itself with the uses and explicit and implicit meanings of food to those who consume it, where food comes from and to whom it goes (and how much), how food can maintain health or prevent disease and behaviours during times of food scarcity and abundance.

However, cultural nutrition goes beyond the bounds of nutritional anthropology, and invites the curious eye of historians, geographers, sociologists, psychologists and folklorists among others. There is certainly a growing cross-disciplinary interest in food habits, as evidenced by a burgeoning body of literature in many fields of study. Indeed, the sheer diversity of sources presents a not inconsiderable challenge to research.

Food choice models

Obviously, the selection of foods by human groups is influenced by a myriad of factors. The answer to the question of why one eats what one eats is indeed a complex one. Most people would probably feel that they are fairly free to choose their own diets, and most people would be surprised to learn the constraints that are in fact operating in limiting their choices. Various models of food choice have been proposed over the years. Some have emphasized environment, others have concentrated on individual motivation. Each has contributed to our understanding of the factors which shape our food choices, while at the same time leaving many questions unanswered. Indeed, it seems unlikely that the plethora of factors which impinge on food choice can be codified in a single paradigm.

Krondl and Boxen (1975) propose a model in which energy is a major determinant of nutritional behaviour. They point out that the diversity of foods available increases along with the growing sophistication of societies, and hypothesize that this is a function of more intense energy inputs. Thus in primitive society food resources were dependent on a combination of solar power and human energy. Agricultural societies could add to these auxiliary energy sources in the form of wind, water and animal power. Industrial societies could further supplement inputs with fossil fuels, hydropower and atomic energy. Increased supplies of energy altered the nature of available food resources by permitting transportation, preservation and technological processing – and thus indirectly influenced nutrition behaviour. At the same time, the authors suggest, decreases in energy required for survival functions has had the effect of largely replacing internal cues to hunger by culturally conditioned external cues. They thus recognize the role of food resources (what they call utility stimuli) and of cultural values (non-utility stimuli) on food behaviour, but posit energy as the underlying determinant. Messer (1984) discusses the limitations of energy models in studying food systems.

Various motivational models are based on the premises that food is symbolic of human values and relationships and that food habits satisfy social needs. In 1943 Kurt Lewin propounded the channel theory, in which he proposed that food moved step by step through 'channels' until it ended up on the table, where it would be eaten by one or other family member. Each of the channels was controlled by a person whom Lewin called the gatekeeper, and who was key to any change efforts. The number of channels and the number of steps within a channel varies for different foods and in different cultural contexts; entrance into and movement through food channels is governed by values such as taste, health, social status and cost. These values interact and actual food choice is thus a complex decision based on motivations of which the consumer may not even be aware. Five decades ago, Lewin was able to consider the housewife as being the gatekeeper of family food intake. With changes in family structures, work opportunities and social roles this can no longer be assumed to be the case. Through in-depth interviews with women of different social classes, Calnan and Fieldhouse (1986) compiled profiles of families and the role that food played in their lives. In most instances it was easy to identify which family member was the dominant influence on the food habits of the family, and that there was a social class difference. Women were most often dominant in higher social class households, whereas men had more influence in lower class households. Childrens' preferences were catered to to a lesser or greater degree but they were rarely the dominant influence on household food choices. Women from higher class households were more likely to put an overall higher priority on food, and to view meal times as a social occasion for all the family to be together, than were their counterparts in the lower class households.

Hierarchy of human needs

Another motivational framework was described by Abraham Maslow (1970) when he applied his well-known human needs model to food usage (Figure 1.1). Maslow classified human needs in terms of physiological and social parameters; he deduced that some needs are more basic than others and was thus able to construct a hierarchy of these needs. He suggested that at least minimum satisfaction of one level of need is required before a person can move up to seek satisfaction of the next higher level of need. Above a minimum level of satisfaction needs may be met to a greater or lesser extent, and progress to the next level is still possible.

Some critics of the Maslow model, while accepting that there are different types of human needs, reject the notion that these are in hierarchical relationship to one another. For example, Duhl (1990) attributes the success of the Sarvodayo movement in Sri Lanka to the fact that it

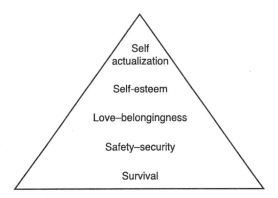

Figure 1.1 Hierarchy of human needs.

attempts to meet different levels of human needs simultaneously. Thus spiritual needs are not neglected in working with hungry people to produce food security. Notwithstanding this, Maslow's hierarchy is presented below as a useful basis for illustrating the biocultural nature of food habits in varying circumstances.

Survival

At the base of the hierarchy are survival needs. No matter what cultural variations exist in food usages, there is one universal imperative; food is fundamental for individual survival. Maslow himself says: 'For the man who is extremely and dangerously hungry, no other interests exist, but food. He dreams food, he remembers food, he thinks food; he emotes only about food, he perceives only food, and he wants only food'. An example of what happens when a group of civilized people are thrust back into a state of survival is provided by an account of the blockade mounted around Leningrad during World War II.

The Siege of Leningrad

In September 1941 German air attacks commenced on the city of Leningrad while ground troops formed a barricade around the city, marking the beginning of a 900-day siege. The people of Leningrad trapped in the blockade were to experience incredible hardships and deprivations, including a drastic reduction of food supplies. Over two-and-a-half million people were trapped in the city, and they had somehow to be fed. Near the beginning of the siege the major food-containing warehouse was destroyed and with it a large part of the city's supply of meat, sugar, butter and grain. Food rationing, which had been imposed earlier in the year, became much more severe and widespread hoarding of food occurred. By November of 1941 deaths from starvation had become commonplace. Desperate people, searching for alternative sources of nourishment, consumed hitherto taboo foods such as dogs, cats and birds. Celluloses such as tree bark and sawdust were added to flour as extenders. 'People began to stuff their stomachs with substitutes. They tore the wallpaper from the walls and scraped off the paste, which was supposed to have been made with potato flour. Some ate the paper. It had nourishment they thought, because it was made from wood. Later they chewed the plaster – just to fill their stomachs.' (Salisbury, 1969).

As the siege continued normal codes of behaviour were increasingly flouted; murder for food or for ration cards became an everyday event. Rumours circulated that human flesh was being used in sausages. Food lines grew and police were authorized to shoot food criminals on the spot. Small amounts of food reached the city across frozen Lake Lagoda, but not until the Spring was there any real relief – when natural greenery provided a source of food. The following year was not so severe due to the reduced number of people to be fed and partial breaks in the blockade, though bombing raids continued to ravage the city. Estimates suggest that between 600 000 and 1 million people died of starvation during the siege.

Security

Once survival needs are assured people begin to worry about food security: that is not just 'will we eat today?' but also 'what will we eat next week?'. Security needs can be met through storage of food. Hoarding of food during a shortage reflects anxiety about this need. The excessive storage of food beyond immediate future needs is common among families in affluent societies, and may be interpreted as a form of insecurity. It is also possible to view some cases of obesity as the result of a security response; parents who have lived through hard times, when food was scarce or rationed, are determined that their offspring will not be similarly deprived, and so overfeed and force food on them. In his classic study of Alorese society, DuBois (1944) suggested that the insecurity which was a dominant personality feature of Alorese adults stemmed from childhood experiences of not having food needs met.

Love–belongingness

When physiological and safety needs are no longer overriding concerns for people, food becomes a way of meeting love, belongingness and affection needs. Food is frequently used to meet such needs, as shown by the use of foods as rewards or gifts or to demonstrate membership of a particular sociocultural group. 'Traditionally, American women have expressed love of family through careful selection, preparation, and service of meals. Accordingly, disparaging remarks about food are tabooed as bad manners. At the same time, a compliment expresses love in a socially acceptable way.' (Eckstein, 1980).

Self-esteem

Self-esteem is next in the hierarchy. Pride in food preparation may be reflective of this and most people enjoy being praised for the quality of the foods they prepare. After the austerity of the Second World War years in Britain, women's magazines began to portray cooking as a source of enjoyment and competitive social display (Mennel, 1985). Lowenberg *et al.* (1979) refer to the popularity of best cook contests in the US. Food manufacturers were quick to exploit this need, presenting advertisements which depict (usually) a housewife receiving praise for her cooking by virtue of having used a particular product. The emphasis is on success and reliability so that tried and true products are to be preferred over individual innovation and experimentation. As the expanding convenience food industry sought new markets, it offered women self-esteem in a can.

Self-actualization

Whereas self-esteem is bolstered through the praise received for the successful preparation of a sure-fire recipe, self-actualization is expressed by the innovative use of foods, new recipes and food experimentation. It only occurs if a person has self-confidence and is not afraid of failure. Self-actualizers dare to be different. Food becomes a personal trademark – a source of personal satisfaction and achievement. Innovative food preparation has long been used as an expression of individual creativity. Historically there have always been plaudits for good chefs, a tradition that is continued undiminished in many parts of the modern world. Chefs who can create beautiful and delicious foods are well rewarded in modern society. Recent years have seen a revival in the art of food preparation, exemplified by an obsession with cook books, magazines and TV chefs. Highly popular, often glossy, magazines stress creativity in cooking, and the majority of their space is devoted to elaborate and aesthetically pleasing dishes. TV chefs command huge viewing audiences and in some instances have practically attained the status of cult figures.

The lower rungs of the hierarchy thus represent predominantly biological needs whereas the upper rungs are more obviously social in nature. Lowenberg *et al.* (1979) contend that most people under normal circumstances try to climb the ladder and that slipping down the ladder signifies a disaster situation. Such may be the case when famine strikes, or during times of severe economic recession. For example, the past decade has seen the emergence in Canada of new institutions known as food banks, which are charitable organizations dedicated to distributing surplus foods to the poor. Loss of employment sends many people tumbling down the rungs of Maslow's hierarchy until they become dependent on the food banks for simply meeting day-to-day needs.

However, what are we to say of instances where individuals actively choose to put themselves back at the lower levels of the hierarchy? For example, the back-to-the-land movement, prominent in the 1960s, saw many people deliberately choosing a simpler lifestyle in which much of their time and energy was devoted to producing enough food just to feed themselves. Is this a case of 'slipping down the ladder'? I think not; rather it represents a form of self-actualization which, paradoxically, resembles the survival stage and in doing so perhaps illustrates the pitfalls of a strict hierarchical view of needs.

Hunger strikes

The drive to obtain food for survival is a fundamental human instinct. When starvation threatens, social behaviour deteriorates as each individual selfishly pursues the quest for food. Because this drive is so powerful it is all the more astonishing to learn of people who deliberately choose to deny themselves food to the point of death. Such action reflects an iron resolve and often stems from an unshakeable belief in certain lauded principles. Thus hunger strikes represent the actions of committed men and women who are willing to die to focus attention on their ideological concerns.

Mahatma Gandhi, that foremost champion of human rights, under-stood the power of self-starvation in drawing attention to his ideas. He made extensive use of hunger strikes – or fasts – which proved to be a potent weapon against the British, and later in reconciling Hindus and Moslems in India. His first public fast was a response to a situation of deadlock between mill-workers and mill-owners at Ahmedabad. Gandhi fasted to keep the mill-workers loyal to their pledge to stay on strike until the owners gave in to their demands; however, his action also put direct pressure on the mill-owners to capitulate as they did not wish to bear responsibility for Gandhi's death. Three days later they accepted arbitration (Fischer, 1950). Gandhi did not fast for personal gain but in order to promote an idea; in this case, the idea of arbitration. In September of 1924 Gandhi fasted in the cause of Hindu–Moslem unity. He had no wish to die but felt that his fast was dictated by his duty to the brotherhood of man. He fasted in the home of a Moslem, thus focusing wide attention on the sight of a Hindu entrusting himself to a Moslem. In 1948 he fasted again in the name of Indian unity – restoring peace to the strife-torn city of Delhi. A full account of this and other Gandhian fasts can be found in Fischer's book.

The use of hunger strikes in attempts to draw attention to political causes is seen in the case of Irish Republican Army prisoners in Northern Ireland. In 1980 there were 39 hunger strikers in the gaols of Northern Ireland. The leading seven strikers in the Maze prison in Belfast were in poor health and determined to die if their demands for special status for Republican prisoners were not met; one of them was losing his eyesight because of a vitamin deficiency; he refused all treatment. The strikers did not attract public sympathy in the way that Gandhi had. Although the British Government hoped that deaths could be avoided it resolved not to give in to what it called blackmail and several hunger strikers subsequently starved to death.

In contrast, in South Africa, in 1989, a spontaneous hunger strike spread among hundreds of people languishing in detention centres. Many had been jailed for months or years without being charged. As the hunger strike spread by word of mouth sympathizers in the outside community also joined in. The authorities, fearing the consequences of any deaths, began releasing prisoners.

Periodically there are reports in the popular media of individual hunger strikes, nearly always designed to draw attention to some perceived injustice either to the individual faster, or on behalf of another group. The deliberate self-denial of food continues to be a powerful demonstration of commitment to an idea or cause.

A FOOD SELECTION PARADIGM

De Garine (1970) suggests that in order to investigate sociocultural aspects of food habits three different parameters have to be measured. First of all come techniques – of food production, storage, distribution, processing and meal preparation. Secondly there is the actual food consumption – including such variables as seasonal fluctuation and status of family members. Finally, attention must be paid to food ideology – how people think about food and its particular meanings and values. Many of these parameters have been incorporated in the various food choice models described earlier. Whichever model of food choice one embraces, one inevitability accepts certain suppositions, prejudices and omissions. Understanding what these limitations are increases the usefulness of the models as tools for study of the real world. The framework presented below recognizes that there are clusters of influences which can be grouped together for convenience of study and which operate at different stages of the food choice process. It does not claim that a particular factor operates exclusively at one level or that all the factors identified have equal importance for all human groups. Table 1.5 depicts a framework built around the twin concepts of availability and acceptability, while Table 1.6 lists some of the component factors in greater detail.

Table 1.5 Food selection paradigm

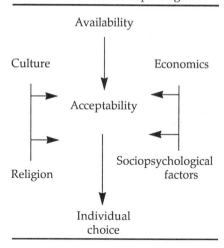

Table 1.6 Elements of food selection

Availability
    Physical

	Political	Economic
Land availability	Agricultural policies	Price
Water availability	Subsidies	Farm costs
Climate	Business controls	Marketing costs
Type of soil	Legislation	Packaging
Pest and plant control	Distribution	Processing
Transportation	Welfare programmes	Transport
Storage facilities	Rationing	Storage
	Nutrition policies	Consumer
	and guidelines	demand
	Government-sponsored	Income
	research activities	
	Trade and aid policies	Patterns
	tariffs and quotas	of expenditure

Acceptability
    Cultural and religious

	Individual choice	Sociopsychological
Ideology	Preference	Prestige
Cuisine	Taste	Status
Myths	Therapeutic needs	Friendship
Superstitions	Personality	Communication
Taboos	Beliefs	Reward and
		punishment
Ritual	Personal values	Emotions
Morals		
Doctrine		
Prohibitions		

Human diets are governed first by what people can get from the environment; given a choice they then eat what their ancestors ate before them (May, 1957). What food is available is a matter of geography and climate, combined with various influences which determine food transportation and distribution capabilities, and policies relating to each of these. Hence physical and political parameters as well as economic ones are of importance. From the universe of foods which are available or potentially available for human consumption a selection is made guided by economic, cultural, sociopsychological and religious rationales. Individual or personal factors come into play after all the other conditions of acceptability have been met. It is in this realm that individual free choice may truly be said to occur, though even here several conditioning factors such as physiological status and therapeutic needs are immediately apparent. It is also worth remembering that personal values, attitudes and beliefs about food, and food preferences are largely shaped during the early socialization period and are thus already a product of culture. The illusion that we choose freely what we eat is perhaps a comforting one, and one which fits into the free will philosophic tradition cherished by millions of people. The truth is that food habits are shaped to a considerable extent by a combination of objective and subjective factors, many of which are beyond individual control.

SUMMARY

The interrelationship of food habits with other elements of cultural behaviour and with environmental forces emphasizes the futility of treating food choices as being intellectual decisions made on rational nutritional grounds alone. Food can be nutritious but not satisfying, and is part of a cultural economy in which material considerations like survival and security are mediated by a philosophical or moral framework. Attempts to change food habits in order to improve nutritional status may be thwarted by failure to understand cultural needs. Where dietary changes are introduced there is the probability that other aspects of social life will also be affected. A corollary to this is that changes in dietary behaviour may be bought about, not by direct modification of food habits, but by alteration or manipulation of the material or non-material culture.

In studying food habits, researchers have developed a number of distinct methodological approaches and have devised several theoretical frameworks in attempts to unify their findings. Food choice models, some of which have been described, are useful in identifying elements of food choice behaviour, but are necessarily incomplete.

FURTHER READING

For an overview of anthropological perspectives on diet and an extensive bibliography, see reference to Messer, 1984.

For a discussion of decision-making processes in relation to personal health and nutrition behaviour, see references to Becker, 1974 and Fieldhouse, 1982.

The work of Frederick Simoons, which is further discussed in Chapters 4 and 6, is an outstanding example of the use of the culture–history approach, as is John Super's enquiry into food, conquest and colonization in Sixteenth-Century Spanish America, (Super, 1988).

A chronology of over 450 famines recorded in historical and literary documents can be found in Keys, A., Brozek, J., Henschel, A., Mickelsen, O., and Taylor, H.L. (1950) *The Biology of Human Starvation*, University of Minneapolis Press, Minneapolis.

Invaluable bibliographies of food and culture have been prepared by Freedman (1981, 1983) and Wilson (1973, 1979), while Grivetti's fascinating work on cultural nutrition themes in art, literature and the humanities also provides a wealth of sources (Grivetti *et al.*, 1987).

DISCUSSION QUESTIONS

1. To what extent are we 'prisoners of our culture' so far as food habits are concerned?
2. How powerful is television as an influence on food habits?
3. Describe the value system of a minority group within your society and suggest how this affects food-related behaviour.
4. The idea of social laggards seems to be analogous to the medical labelling of individuals as non-compliers; both imply recalcitrance or failure, which can be overcome if only enough 'education' can be applied. From another perspective, non-compliers and laggards may be seen as non-conformists or resisters who choose to place their own needs goals and values above those of the social engineers and health professionals. Discuss these opposing notions using nutritional illustrations.

LITERATURE SOURCES FOR THE STUDENT OF CULTURAL NUTRITION

Nutrition and cross-disciplinary journals

Annual Review of Anthropology
Annual Review of Nutrition
Current Anthropology

Ecology of Food and Nutrition
Ethnobiology
Food and Nutrition Bulletin of the United Nations
Food and Foodways
Food Policy
Human Ecology
Journal of the American Dietetic Association
Journal of Interdisciplinary History
Journal of Nutrition Education
Medical Anthropology
Nutrition Research
Social Science and Medicine
Social Science Information
World Review of Nutrition and Dietetics

Computer data-bases

AGRICOLA National Agricultural Library, Beltsville
ERIC National Institute of Education, Washington DC
MEDLINE United States National Library of Medicine, Bethesda
PAIS INTERNATIONAL Public Affairs Information Service, New York
SOCIAL SCISEARCH Institute for Scientific Information, Philadelphia
SOCIOLOGICAL ABSTRACTS Sociological Abstracts Inc., San Diego

CHAPTER 2

Food ideology

Just as there are political ideologies which express beliefs concerning how people ought to behave in social relationships, so there are food ideologies which explain how they are to conduct themselves with regard to eating behaviour. Food ideology is the sum of the attitudes, beliefs and customs and taboos affecting the diet of a given group. It is what people think of as food; what effect they think food will have on their health and what they think is suitable for different ages and groups (Eckstein, 1980). Sometimes, the most surprising items emerge as food. Was it Ogden Nash's pioneer who first thought of trying to eat artichokes? (Nash, 1968); whoever decided that raw oysters or rotting game were delicacies?, and who was persistent enough to entrench red-hot chili peppers as a firm favourite in the diet? The very idea of acquired taste indicates that there are foods which are not intrinsically appealing and which we have to actively learn to enjoy.

While it seems that some unusual dietary choices have been made by various human groups it is also true that of all of the animal and vegetable substances which could serve as human food only a few are selected for actual consumption; that is, certain potential foodstuffs are rejected because they are not acceptable. What is deemed to be acceptable constitutes an important part of the cultural stability of a society and is passed on from generation to generation via the socialization process. An idea of how we quickly categorize foods according to ethnocentric rules of acceptability can be gained by asking yourself 'Would I eat these foodstuffs?'.

- Cereals (wheat? – corn? – millet?)
- Fruit (apple? – lime? – mango?)
- Milk (cow's? – goat's? – sheep's?)
- Meat (Beef? – pork? – horse? – dog? – raw meat?)
- Insects

All of the above are potential foodstuffs. Millet, a staple in many African countries is rejected as 'bird seed' in richer countries. Milk evokes feelings of disgust in some societies. Meat-eaters will eat only certain kinds of meat. Westerners may be revolted at the thought of eating insects. The point is that no social group classifies as food all the potential foodstuffs which are available. Moreover, where there is more than sufficient food available for survival, choices are made which are assertions of identity (Back, 1977). In the same ecological environment with similar technological resources at their disposal different societies will make different choices among the available resources. For example in Senegal, the Serer and Wolof tribes use all parts of the baobob tree – yet 4000 km away in climatically similar Chad, only the fruit is used (de Garine, 1976).

ETHNOCENTRISM

Ethnocentrism describes the belief that one's own patterns of behaviour are preferable to those of all other cultures. Because people are taught the values of the culture in which they grow up they tend to view their own patterns of behaviour as being right, normal and best. As a corollary to this, foreign cultures are viewed as being wrong or irrational or misguided. So engrained are such attitudes that some degree of ethnocentrism is virtually inescapable, though exposure to other cultures can broaden tolerance and aid in an understanding of how other peoples live.

Food habits are an integral part of cultural behaviour and are often closely identified with particular groups, sometimes in a derogatory or mocking way. So, the French are 'Frogs', the Germans are 'Krauts', the Italians are 'Spaghetti eaters' and the British, 'Limeys'. The word 'Eskimo' is an Indian word meaning 'eaters of raw flesh', and was originally used to express the revulsion of one group toward the food habits of another. Eskimos refer to themselves as 'Inuit', which literally means 'real people' – and is itself a linguistic example of ethnocentrism, implying as it does that members of other societies are not 'real people'. The Toupouri of Northern Cameroon ritually eat rotting legs of beef and for that are mocked by their neighbours, the Moussey, who are in return derided by the Toupouri for their habit of using the juice of centipedes in sauces. Food ridicule can be considered as one of the criteria determining the boundaries of a culture (de Garine 1976). Exposure to unfamiliar food habits is almost guaranteed to bring ethnocentrism to the fore. At an informal supper I once attended in Alberta, the beef capital of Canada, lamb was served (albeit in the form of lamb-burgers). Most of the people present took some convincing even to try this strange meat; those who did were surprised to find it to be quite acceptable. One confirmed lamb-eater, an Irishman, was mercilessly teased (or ridiculed) for his preference, and the attitude of the group was summed up by one member who asked why anyone should want to eat lamb when there was beef available.

Sometimes people will quite happily eat a food until they discover what it is that they are eating, when they suddenly become quite ill. Thus it is the idea of what is food, as much as the food itself, which evokes both physiological and psychological feelings. Ogden Nash captures this feeling perfectly in one of his poems entitled 'Experiment Degustatory'. After overcoming initial feelings of disgust, the hero of the poem discovers that rattlesnake meat tastes just like chicken; unfortunately he is subsequently unable to face the thought of eating chicken – because it tastes like rattlesnake meat! (Nash, 1968). Probably everyone has had this kind of experience at one time or another, perhaps with less exotic delicacies than rattlesnake meat. The feelings aroused by the sudden knowledge that one is eating octopus rather than fish or that the tasty jugged hare on one's plate is actually guinea pig can cause one to pause in mid-bite, or to make a hurried dash for the bathroom. The actual flavour of the food is irrelevant, for we don't even have to taste a food to label it as unacceptable or disgusting; our culture tells us what is fit to eat, and our ethnocentricity ensures that we obey.

CULTURAL RELATIVISM

Cultural relativism is an approach to understanding cultures which attempts to overcome the in-built prejudices of ethnocentrism. In this conceptual framework cultural practices must be examined within the context of the indigenous cultural group; if they are not dysfunctional within that group then they must be accepted as normal, no matter how different they be from our own familiar practices. Cultural relativism in effect says that there aren't really any universal standards of behaviour against which everybody should be judged. However, some values are very widely shared across cultures; for example, most societies have sanctions against indiscriminate killing and other persistent anti-social behaviour. Nevertheless, the ability to set aside one's own cultural biases and preferences helps significantly in understanding the food practices and values of other societies. If we appreciate this then we may not be quite so ready to dismiss as irrational the Sacred Cow taboo of Hinduism, or to reject as disgusting the eating of insects and grubs. We may also realize that our own food practices could seem irrational or disgusting from the vantage point of another culture. What, for example, are we to make of a pet-loving society which spends huge amounts of money on food and care for animals which themselves have no value as human food, or the sportsman who hangs game birds until they begin to rot?

FOOD CATEGORIZATION

In every society, there are rules – usually unwritten – which specify what is food and what is not. Within the larger classification of 'food', subgroups or categories of foodstuffs are identified according to nutritional value, cultural usage, emotional importance, or a combination thereof. In fact, there are numerous ways of classifying or categorizing foods and food usages. Sometimes the classifications have an obvious rational basis; some, with less apparent rationality, have grown out of coherent folk-medicine systems; yet others are a result of mere fancy or caprice. Many of these reflect the rational needs or ethnocentric views of the classifiers, and it may be difficult to justify their existence in reality.

Eckstein (1980) uses the concept of 'food or poison' to divide what is eaten from what is not. Whatever is not defined as food is automatically poison, an idea which suggests that the adage 'one man's meat is another man's poison' is literally true. There are several perspectives from which the food/poison classification can be made. Eckstein lists the following, most of which are discussed in later chapters. Physiological; Emotional/psychological; Sociocultural; Health-related; Economic; Aesthetic; Sub-group.

Once we have differentiated 'food' from 'poison' we proceed to assign values based on a variety of possible criteria. For centuries, different cultures have divided foods into varying numbers of categories based on their actual or imagined properties or on their supposed effect on the body or on disease processes. Ancient Chinese physicians identified four food categories, each with five foods, that they deemed especially nourishing to the body and useful when treating disease (Grivetti, 1991c). The Indian document known as the Caraka-Samhita, from around 1500 BCE, lists 12 food groups (Grivetti, 1991a)(Table 2.1).

Table 2.1 Ancient food categories*

China	
Grains:	beans; millet; peas, rice, wheat
Fruits:	almonds/apricots; chestnuts, dates; peaches; plums
Vegetables:	greens; leeks; mallows; onions; scallions
Domesticated animals:	chicken; dog; lamb; pig; ox
India	
Grains	
Legumes	
Meats	
Vegetables	
Fruits	
Salads and greens	
Alcoholic beverages	
Rain water	
Milk and milk products	
Sweeteners	
Combination dishes and products	
Condiments	

*Adapted from Grivetti, L.E. (1991a) Nutrition Past – Nutrition Today. Prescientific Origins of Nutrition and Dietetics. *Nutrition Today*, Part 1, Jan/Feb, p.21; Part 3, Nov/Dec, p.11.

Perhaps the categorization most familiar to nutritionists today and which is perpetuated through formal instruction and printed materials, is the one in which foods are classified according to nutritional value. This is the basis for food guides such as the Food Guide Pyramid in the US, Canada's Food Guide to Healthy Eating, and the Food Groups of the UK National Dairy Council. In each case, the categories are designed to facilitate the choice of nutritionally balanced diets within the framework of normal cultural eating patterns. Usually, a food group includes a selection of foodstuffs rich in a particular nutrient or nutrients; by combining foods from each group a wide spectrum of nutrients is obtained, thereby ensuring nutritional adequacy. Food groups are basically a nutritionist's teaching tool and do not seem to reflect the way in which people actually do classify their own foods. Although students are taught, and eagerly take up, the use of food guides, few of them can honestly say that that is how they choose their own food intake. Moreover, food guides, far from being objectively based on the latest scientific knowledge, are at least in part a reflection of changing political economies and, to a greater or lesser degree, are shaped to meet the desires of powerful interest groups. The fact that food groups differ between countries which accept broadly the same nutritional understanding and goals also shows that they are a cultural construct.

As chronic disease and health promotion have replaced deficiency diseases as a major cause of nutritional concern the basic message of variety has become more complex, introducing the ideas of proportionality and moderation. US food guides have changed over the years to reflect regional, then national and now global food patterns of production and consumption. As the production of food has shifted from subsistence and home farming to commerce and multinational agribusiness, the language of food guides has changed from foods to nutritional deficiencies to nutritional excesses. Food Guides, says Lindenbaum (1986), are not innocent categories. 'They are the coded reflections and agendas of social groups organized to influence the political, economic and cultural life of different generations of producers, distributors and consumers'.

Similarly, revisions to the Canada Food Guide were heavily influenced by industry lobby groups, particularly the meat and dairy sectors. Modifications aimed at reducing the total fat content of the diet, including fewer and smaller servings of meat, were resisted vigorously. One popular media commentator remarked that the 'four food groups' should perhaps be called the 'four food interest groups'. In 1992 Canada's Food Guide evolved from a long-standing circle depiction to a rainbow graphic which, while retaining the same four food groups, tried to depict visually the ideas of proportionality. This qualitative tool was combined with a quantitative list of recommended servings for different age and physiological population groups. In addition, the guide attempted to incorporate broader health promotion messages such as active living and enjoyment of life, encapsulated by the slogan 'Vitality'. In response to critiques of cultural hegemony in the food guide, foods were depicted which it was felt would find broad acceptance among diverse ethnic groups. Further adaptations to meet specific cultural needs were left to the discretion and creativity of local practitioners. The government of the North West Territories had already recognized the deficiencies of a national food guide based on southern urban eating habits and in 1988, in conjunction with the Medical Services Branch of Health and Welfare Canada, produced a version utilizing northern foods and printed in the Inuktitut language (Figure 2.1).

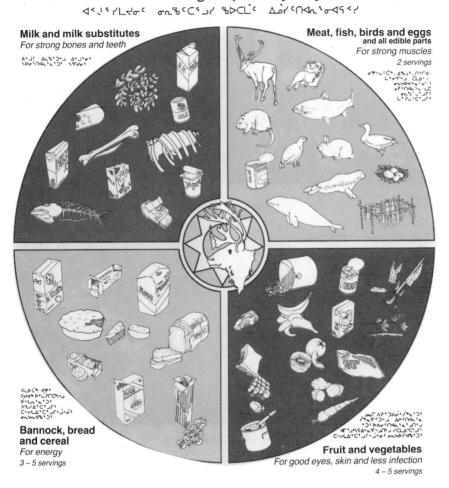

N.W.T. FOOD GUIDE

ᓄᓇ� ᑦᓯᐊᕐᒥ ᓂᕿ� ᑲᑐᒃ Lᑭᒃᐸᒃᑲ

Eat foods from each group every day for Health

ᐊᑨᒋᕐᒥᒃᑐᒃ ᓂᕐᖃᑦᑕᒥ ᖃᐅᒻᑖᓴ ᐄᓇᕐᒃᕿᓐᖓᑨᐊᕿᖅ

Milk and milk substitutes
For strong bones and teeth

Meat, fish, birds and eggs
and all edible parts
For strong muscles
2 servings

Bannock, bread and cereal
For energy
3 – 5 servings

Fruit and vegetables
For good eyes, skin and less infection
4 – 5 servings

Figure 2.1 North-West Territories food guide.

National food guides tend to be based largely on rationalist scientific assumptions, though more recent versions acknowledge the importance of customary eating patterns, personal acceptability and cultural variation. Other classification systems recognize the interaction between biological and cultural factors. For example; Bass, Wakefield and Kolassa (1979) suggest that people classify food according to: its actual use by the body; its actual use in society; its perceived use by the body and in society. In this scheme, potatoes are used as: a source of energy and minerals for the body; a food for snacks and meals; perceived as being 'fattening' and a filler food for meals. The authors do not elaborate on this classification or demonstrate how it might be used in practice, though it seems to suggest a multi-stage process whereby a particular food is judged to be appropriate or non-appropriate by a series of criteria. Let's say we were considering choosing an egg for breakfast; first of all it is a good source of protein; secondly, it is an appropriate food for this meal; lastly, it is judged to give us a good start to the day (Witness the British Egg Marketing Board's 'Go to work on an egg' advertising slogan). The egg is therefore accepted.

One of the limitations of food taxonomies is that categories are usually derived from the perspective of the researcher rather than that of the consumer. Schutz, Rucker and Russell (1975) asked people to express their own judgements about foods and as a result found four common food-use factors: utilitarian, casual, satiating and social. They also reported consumer classifications of actual foods as falling into five main categories:

1. High calorie treats.
   Cakes and pies figured prominently in this category of foods considered appropriate for social occasions. Snacks such as celery or carrot sticks were deemed to be more suitable for when eating alone; they were more 'everyday'.
2. Speciality meal items.
   Only to be served in particular circumstances, and definitely not everyday foods. Some foods placed in this category (e.g. chilli) are everyday foods for other ethnic groups.
3. Common meal items.
   Foods served at the dinner meal and seen to be suitable for all occasions and all ages. Meats ranked high in this category.
4. Refreshing foods.
   Foods such as milk and orange juice were regarded as suitable for serving cold – though not as an entrée. They were thought to be nutritious and easy to digest.
5. Inexpensive filling foods.
   These were often high calorie, but lacked the social function or prestige of foods in category 1. Thus, bread, potato chips (crisps), chocolate bars

and peanut butter appeared in this category. They were regarded as being unsuitable when weight loss was desired.

Although the actual categories were created by the authors on the basis of consumer responses, and are thus the product of scientific interpretation, it is interesting to note that a biological basis for classification is less readily discernable than in the previously described systems. Nor is this particularly surprising. The majority of people, even those with extensive schooling, do not have a firm grasp of the nutritional value of foodstuffs. What they do understand, is the cultural meaning and usage of food – and people make decisions based on what they know. Thus whereas those educated in nutritional principles can appreciate the scientific rationality of food groups, those without such training follow other indicators. The verity and utility of classifications such as that of Schutz *et al.* may certainly be questioned, but they at least merit further study as potential 'popular' tools for teaching sound nutrition.

Messer (1984) comments that with the possible exception of modern Western society, no cultural group evaluates the individual foods and combinations which it ingests in terms of the scientific categories of energy, fat, protein, vitamins and minerals. Most commonly, foods are assigned values according to their functional role as well as their perceived nutritional and non-nutritional effects. Derek Jelliffe, who is noted for his cross-cultural studies in nutrition, offers the following 'world-wide' classification system; cultural superfoods, prestige foods, body-image foods, sympathetic magic foods, physiologic group foods (Jelliffe, 1967). Cultural superfoods are the dominant staple foods of a society. Much effort is expended in producing and preparing them and they are often involved in the religious rituals and the mythology of the society. Prestige foods are those reserved for important occasions or for important people. They are characterized by relative scarcity and high price. Body-image foods are those which contribute to good health by maintaining a balance in the body. Yin–yang and hot–cold food dichotomies (discussed below) are examples of systems which embody this idea. In Western culture we hold the idea of fattening and slimming foods. Sympathetic magic foods are those which are believed to have special properties which are imparted to those who eat them. Physiological group foods are foods restricted to persons of a particular age, sex or physiological condition.

As in the food selection paradigm presented in Chapter 1, the contribution of religion, economics, and sociocultural factors in shaping food behaviour is clearly shown by this classification. The purpose of food categorization is often a descriptive one – to reveal how foods are assigned value in a society, whereas for the nutritionist or dietitian concerned with promoting healthy eating habits prescriptive categories are obviously more attractive, as they can be used to advise others on how food choices should be made. One approach which goes some way toward addressing both these needs comes from the early work of Passim and Bennett (1943) and is still useful today when considering strategies of dietary change. Dietary intake is divided into three categories of core, secondary and peripheral items in order to distinguish the frequency of consumption and the importance given to various foods.

Core foods are universal, regular, staple, important and consistently used foods. Most members of the society will use these foods, which form the mainstay of the diet. Resistance to dietary modification will be greatest with reference to these core items. Examples would be cereal staples; large portions of meat in Northern cultures; milk, potatoes and bread. Secondary foods are in widespread but not universal use; they may be thought of as supporting actors, playing differing roles in the diet. They are of less emotional importance to most people, and include recently introduced, and store-bought foods. Changes in respect of secondary items are more readily accepted. Most fruits and vegetables probably fall into this category, as do items such as cake mixes and tinned soups. Peripheral foods are least common and are infrequently consumed. They may be new foods or items only included through economic necessity. Their use is characteristic of individuals, and they are most amenable to change with the least of emotional resistance. Oysters and offal (sweetbreads) might be two very different examples of items in this category. Of course, what are peripheral foods for most people in a culture might be of greater importance to the few.

Analysis of a patient's diet in terms of core, secondary and peripheral foods would provide the wary dietitian with an indication of where dietary modifications could be most readily made and where resistance might be anticipated. Such analyses could also add to our understanding of the phenomenon of non-compliance with dietary regimes. (Non-compliance may also be interpreted as a decision to put personal needs before goals of the professional.)

Another prescriptive system of food classification which is in widespread use in certain cultural traditions and in folk medicine in Northern countries is one based on principles of allopathic medicine. Because it is a popular concept in folk medicine and because it represents an alternative way of assessing food values, the origins, development and modern practice of allopathy is discussed at some length below.

Dietary systems and allopathic medicine

Allopathy is an ancient system of treatment by opposites which is still practised in many parts of the world today. Foods, diseases and parts of the body are assigned various attributes, notably hot–cold valences. Disease is said to occur when the body is out of balance and balance is restored by treating a cold illness with hot or heating foods and vice versa.

The system is endlessly elaborated and may incorporate several other dimensions in addition to hot–cold. Allopathy probably originated in India sometime in the second millennium BCE from where it spread eastwards to China and westwards to the Mediterranean and subsequently, via European explorers to the Americas. It became entrenched in the folk medicine of diverse cultures and today is common in Latin America, India, China, North Africa and the Caribbean. In North America, allopathy thrives among immigrant Hispanic, Asian and Mediterranean populations.

Origins in India

The traditional healing system of India is known as Ayurvedic medicine, from the eternal knowledge or ayurveda which was passed from Brahma the creator, to humans. The ayurvedic dietary system is based on three concepts, familiar to modern scientific nutritionists: assessment of clinical signs and symptoms; acknowledgement that behaviour and environment influences health or disease; belief that proper food and diet restores health. Health is a sign of balance in the body and is compromised when imbalance occurs in one or more of the elements, humours, organ feeders or tastes (Table 2.2).

Table 2.2 Indian Ayurvedic system

Elements (bhutas)	Humours (dosas)	Organ feeders (dhātus)	Tastes (rasas)
Earth (prithive)		Organic juice (rasa)	Sweet (madhura)
Water (appu)	Water (kapha)	Blood (raka)	Sour (amla)
Fire (theyu)	Fire (pitta)	Flesh (mamsa)	Salt (lavana)
Air/wind (vayu)	Air (vayu)	Fat (medas)	Pungent (katu)
Ether (akasa)		Bone (asthi)	Bitter (katu)
		Marrow (majja)	Astringent (kashaya)
		Semen (sukra)	

Anna, or food, is the life principle and all foods are compounded of five bhutas or elements; earth, water, fire, air and ether. The human body is also made up of these elements, which are associated with the five senses. Foods also have six taste qualities (sweet, sour, salt, pungent, bitter, astringent) one of which is dominant in a given food. Different proportions of the five elements determine the taste of a specific food, which in turn is related to metabolic processes in the body. Food is digested and converted to basic juice (rasa) which turns into six dhātus; blood, flesh, fat, bone, marrow, and semen and into seven secondary body elements including mother's milk and menstrual blood. Digestion of food and metabolism of dhātus produces both prasāda, the nutritive power of food, and mala, the polluting or waste elements (Rao, 1986). The three most important waste products are the humours known as vayu or dosas (air or wind), pitta (fire or bile) and kapha (water or phlegm). Humoural balance is achieved by management of the six tastes, which in turn are balanced through proper dietary selections. Three tastes increase one humour while three different tastes decrease the same humour (Table 2.3). Finally, each taste possesses one or other of a series of dichotomized properties; hot/cold, heavy/light, oily/dry; mild/sharp; compact/mobile; soft/hard; clean/slimy; smooth/rough; minute/gross; solid/liquid. Three common foods, oil, ghee and honey are perceived to be especially therapeutic in restoring humoural balance. Oil, which is hot, heavy and smoothing, counters air humour which is cold, light and rough. Ghee, which is cold, dull and sweet balances fire humour which is hot, sharp and sour. Honey, which is astringent, rough and sharp complements water humour which is sweet, smoothing and dull.

Table 2.3 Relationship of the six tastes to the three humours in the Ayurvedic system

Humour		Tastes
Air	Increased by:	Astringent; bitter; pungent
	Decreased by:	Salty; sweet; sour
Fire	Increased by:	Pungent; salty; sour
	Decreased by:	Astringent; bitter; sweet
Water	Increased by:	Salty; sour; sweet
	Decreased by:	Astringent; bitter; pungent

Diseases, caused by imbalance in one or more of the bhutas, dhātus or dosas could range from mild to chronic and were treated by prescription of proper proportions of wholesome foods. Given that cooking techniques, seasonality, and geographical source could also affect the characteristics of foods, practitioners had at their disposal an almost unlimited range of permutations of different specific foods and food combinations in applying the allopathic principles of opposites.

Modern-day Southern Asia

Modern-day Asian beliefs regarding hot and cold vary between countries and regions; for example, while eggs are perceived as cooling foods in Thailand, they are hot in Bangladesh. Katona-Apte (1977), describing food habits in Tamilnad, says hot and cold classifications vary even with individuals. In Hindu society, raw foods are hot and therefore purer than cooked foods which are cold – a dichotomy which has repercussions within the caste system where it delimits food preparation and sharing practices (Hasan, 1971). In Bangladesh, foods are categorized as strength-giving, blood-producing, hot or cold, nirdosh–nirog, and bitter. Good health means having enough blood, a source of strength and energy. Fish is blood-producing (if it itself has blood), while ghee and milk top the list of strength-giving foods. Bangalis believe that one cannot feel strong without eating rice (Rizvi, 1986). Nirdosh means harmless, and nirog means disease-free; these are neutral foods which do not cause any disease and which do not upset humoural balance in body. Most non-leafy green vegetables are considered nirdosh. Bitter tasting vegetables keep the blood clean and protect from skin infection and intestinal worms – though they are not categorized as being nutritious.

In the Indian region of South Kanara, foods are classified on the basis of multiple criteria and in accord with different levels of analysis. Nichter (1986) says that few villagers are familiar with the principles of āyurveda though they use the terminology, and that food classifications, while not of great concern in everyday life, become of greater importance during illness. As well as hot–neutral–cold and tri dosa (humoural) classifications, villagers also put foods into five other food categories on the basis of perceived or experienced physiological effects: (i) Nañju foods are difficult to digest but also aggravate existing poisons in the blood; (ii) Uri Śīta foods are cooling in nature but cause a heating reaction in body; (iii) Dhātu foods are strength and health-giving; (iv) Uri nañju foods cause watery diarrhoea; and (v) Jedda foods are difficult to digest. In addition, some foods are Hula dośa and cause worm trouble.

Physiological signs and symptoms are ascribed to a food post hoc, sometimes after quite an interval, and there are idiosyncratic food classifications based on differences in individual experiences with eating a food. As well as being classified according to perceived effects foods are also classed according to a wide variety of physical, sensory and situational properties including physical appearance, colour, taste, smell, habitat, domestication, season of harvest, stage of ripeness, water content, mode of preparation and food combinations (Table 2.4).

Table 2.4 Food categories used in South Kanara

Physical appearance
        Shape, texture and consistency of a food may cause it to be classified as similar to other foods which it resembles. e.g. fleshy mushrooms are compared to meat and therefore not eaten by vegetarians
Colour
        Green and white is associated with coolness; red, orange and yellow with heat. White is also associated with easy digestion
Taste
        Six tastes affect body humours in particular ways. Tastiness is also indication of food quality
Smell
        The most important smell is hasi, or rawness and the smell of raw vegetables is often considered intolerable and thought to cause indigestion
Habitat
        Food qualities are associated with the dry/wet, hot/cold qualities of the region where it is grown, and also with the type of soil and fertilizer
Domestication
        Wild foods are qualitatively differentiated from domesticated foods, being considered to have greater dhātu potential and medicinal properties
Season of harvest
        Food takes on the quality of the season; e.g. monsoon rice is cooler than second-crop winter rice. Some foods are thought to change qualities with the season
Stage of ripeness
        The process of ripening is associated with increased heat. Fruition is associated with relative coolness
Water content
        Foods with greater water content are often classified as cooling
Mode of preparation
        Frying increases the heating qualities of food – boiling reduces heat
Mixed preparation
        Qualities of food may be transformed when combined with other foods – this underlies popular recipes for reducing unwanted characteristics of particular foods

---

Adapted from Nichter, M. (1986) Modes of Food Classification and the Diet–Health Contingency: A South Indian Case Study, in *Food, Society, and Culture: Aspects in South Asian Food Systems*, (eds R.S. Khare and M.S.A Rao), Carolina Academic Press, Durham, pp. 185–222.

Mediterranean connections

The writings of Hippocrates demonstrate well-developed allopathic medical nutritional approaches to treatment quite unlike those of Egypt, Carthage or Phoenicia. Grivetti suggests that they parallel Indian concepts and speculates that it was Ctesias, a contemporary of

Hippocrates who had visited India and worked extensively in Persia, who introduced allopathic principles to Greek medicine.

Greek humoural theory held that there were four bodily elements each of which had particular characteristics: blood – hot and wet; phlegm – cold and wet; black bile – cold and dry; yellow bile – hot and dry. Medical practice consisted of understanding the normal mixture of humours or complexion of a person, the complexion of their illness and the method of restoring harmony in the body. Health was also influenced by age, climate, weather, season and lifestyle. Three hundred years after Hippocrates, Celsus of Verona wrote extensively on allopathic nutrition. He believed that certain categories of food were stronger than others, hinting at differences in caloric and protein content. Celsus prescribed diets that balanced nine descriptive attributes assigned to foods. Foods produced 'good juice or bad'; were bland or acrid; thickened or reduced phlegm; were suitable or alien to the stomach; were hot or cold; were easily or poorly digested; were laxative or constipating; were diuretic; promoted sleep or excited the senses. The allopathic legacy was continued by Jewish, Christian and Moslem physicians into the Middle Ages. Avicenna, the famous medieval Moslem physician wrote texts that form the basis of modern Mediterranean allopathic practices.

To the New World

Mediterranean allopathic concepts formed the core of Iberian practice during the Middle Ages and were carried to the New World during the period of European exploration and colonization. The Spaniards established medical teaching at the University of Mexico in 1580 where they taught the principles of humoural medicine. However, early written accounts show that hot–cold concepts pre-existed within the Aztec civilization well before the arrival of the Spaniards in 1519. The Aztecs used 18 sets of paired terms to structure the world, including hot–cold. Of the 18 terms, six were similar to those used in Mediterranean allopathy, but 14 paralleled the Chinese pattern (see below). This has led some scholars to suggest that Europeans were not the first to encounter New World Americans.

The Spanish legacy flourished in Mexico, eventually extending throughout Central and South America and into the south-west United States. Because of the relative isolation of the region, these ideas persisted for longer than in Europe and became firmly embedded in traditional medicine. 'A large component of present day Latin American folk medicine relies on the concept of emotional experiences – shame, fear, anger, envy – as causes of illness, and probably survives from pre-Conquest belief' (Sanjur, 1982).

In Latin American allopathy we once again encounter the notion that health is a temperate condition and that a balance between hot and cold elements must be maintained. Although the body as a whole is temperate, specific parts of it may vary in degree of hotness or coldness; intestines and stomach are hot, mouth and throat are cold. Blood is hot, milk is cold. Most groups practising this lore agree that an excess of cold is more dangerous than an excess of hot; hot foods are easier to digest because the stomach is hot, while cold foods have to be heated by the stomach before they can be digested. Food mixtures and combinations should produce an overall temperate effect, and so meals are to be carefully constructed to avoid extremes. Hot–cold properties of foods are not always constant. Molony (1975) discusses Mexican hot–cold valences, pointing out, in a way reminiscent of Nichter's South Indian study, that they are based on perceived qualities of foods; how a plant was grown, what an animal ate, how a food was cooked, how foods were combined. Chickens are hot if they eat a lot of raw corn; maize corn is hot – because plants needs little water, but becomes cold if boiled in water. (Andeans also believe that exposure to water changes the temperature rating of foods. Usually, the effect of cooking is to moderate ratings.) The hot–cold concept is stronger in Latin America than it ever was in Spain. Therefore, says Sanjur, it must serve some useful function as a basis for preventive and curative folk medicine. Indeed, pellagra – which is a cold illness – is treated by giving hot foods, including peanuts which are high in niacin, the B-vitamin which is deficient in the diet of pellagrins. With this example, Logan (1972) points out how modern medicine can take advantage of traditional belief systems by building on current accepted practices.

The Chinese connection

From its origins in ancient India, allopathic practice spread east to China and found expression in the yin–yang principle. The concept of yin and yang pervades all aspects of traditional Chinese life. Yin is female, dark, wet and cold while yang is male, light, dry and hot. These attributes are applied to foods and to diseases and must be balanced to produce harmony.

The alignment between the yin–yang dichotomy and the five elements of water, fire, wood, metal and earth is central to Chinese medical and dietary treatment. All diseases are designated yin or yang. All foods are yin, yang or neutral. Both disease and food categories are changeable depending on such things as season, geographical location and method of cooking. Disease states are influenced by a specific element, planet, season, climate, direction and number; food attributes and properties are defined by a specific colour, taste and smell; specific animals and plants also are aligned. Parts of the body, whether hollow or solid organs, sense organs, tissues or body orifices, are identified with strong or weak yin, neutrality, strong or weak yang. In addition, body secretions, human attributes and emotions are aligned. Disease occurs when the body becomes imbalanced and energy cannot circulate. Diseases caused by improper diet appear initially in the spleen and are diagnosed by characteristic dietary cravings for specific flavours. Each disease, whether classified yin or yang is also hot or cold and sometimes wet or dry. Grivetti comments that the Chinese system is more complicated and sophisticated than its Indian or Mediterranean counterparts.

Reproduction

In all cultures practising allopathy, the hot–cold concept is closely tied to the reproductive cycle. Imbalances must be particularly avoided by menstruating, pregnant and lactating women. Examples follow from Latin American, South Asian and Chinese practice. For Latin Americans, menstruation is a warm condition so that cold foods – which cause cramps – must be avoided. Infertility is caused by a cold womb and is cured by heating it with tea made from hot herbs. Pregnancy is warm, so cold foods are avoided because of increased vulnerability to cold at this time. Bolivian peasants prohibit cold foods during pregnancy and lactation (de Esquef, 1972). Puerto Rican women, studied by Harwood (1971) considered pregnancy to be a hot state, and avoided hot foods and medications in order to prevent babies from being born with a rash or a red skin. Some women would avoid vitamin and iron supplements which were also considered to be hot. In Chinese practice, non-pregnant women are yin but when they become pregnant they are strongest yang. This shift is paralleled by a dramatic changes in diet. During the hottest yang of pregnancy women must eat yin foods – strict adherence to which can produce low birth-weight babies. Cultural encouragement of yin foods is associated with fewer delivery complications associated with small female body frames.

Latin American women refer to the 40 days following childbirth as 'la cuerenta' or 'la dieta'. At birth, the foetus takes a great deal of warmth from the mother and so a post-partum woman is warmly wrapped and avoids cold foods. Hot foods are prescribed to diminish post-partum bleeding. Similarly in Chinese tradition hot foods are recommended post-partum to stimulate blood and prevent anaemia. During the post-partum period the mother's state changes to strongest yin and she should now base her diet on yang foods. Since yang foods typically are those higher in energy and protein this shift is a cultural way to provide biologically for increased milk production requirements. For the first 6 days after childbirth Bangladeshi women are expected to follow a broad set of dietary rules. The mother is believed to be in her coldest state and restrictions are imposed to aid the healing process and protect the mother from disease. Water is also restricted and must be boiled to remove its coldness which might make the mother susceptible to cold and fever. The end of the post-partum period is celebrated on the sixth day by a special meal of rice, fish and some harmless greens, the purpose being to reduce the mother's food restrictions and introduce the baby (via breast milk) to a wide variety of foods. It is also an occasion to celebrate the survival of the mother and baby. In the late post-partum period emphasis shifts from proscription to prescription. Eating of blood-producing fish is highly recommended to regain lost strength. After 40 days post-partum the hot–cold dichotomy is not ordinarily observed, but the value of strength-giving and blood-producing foods continues to be emphasized (Rizvi, 1986).

In Latin American practice, during lactation heat is believed to increase the supply of milk while cold diminishes it. Too much warmth within the mother may displace cold and concentrate it in the breast causing the milk to curdle and become indigestible. The implications of this are that when a second pregnancy is diagnosed (pregnancy is a hot condition) the nursing child should be immediately weaned in order to forestall problems of curdled milk. As in the case of food withdrawal because of sickness, cessation of breast feeding without adequate substitutes for breast milk may give rise to malnutrition (Sanjur, 1974). In Chinese practice, lactating women should avoid cold and raw foods, alcohol and salt. For Bangali mothers breast milk is considered to be cool or temperate and is disease-free and many women especially in rural areas also categorize powdered milk as a cool disease-free food.

An example of physiological consequences of food classification is found in the ranking of animal milks in terms of their heating effects. In India, animal milk is generally considered to be heating and therefore a danger to infant health if undiluted. Consequent dilution with water may give rise to problems of malnutrition if the mixture is too thin to provide adequate protein and energy. Further, when a child develops infective diarrhoea which is a hot illness, hot foods such as milk are withdrawn completely and the diet changes to one of cool foods such as barley water, a practice which may contribute to development of kwashiorkor. However, it is also true that carbohydrate intolerance is frequently associated with diarrhoea; high carbohydrate loads aggravate the problem and their removal from the diet may actually be beneficial. (In addition, malabsorption syndrome, related to decreased levels of intestinal lactase is not uncommon in Asia.) Buffalo's milk, cow's milk and goat's milk are ranked in a descending order of heat and are consequently diluted more or less to make them suitable for infant feeding. The different heats match the differing lactose contents of the milks; thus those milks with higher lactose concentrations, and which are therefore more likely to cause problems of intestinal malabsorption, are diluted more (McCracken, 1971).

Variance in classification of foods

Interpretation of the hot–cold system is made difficult in view of the fact that there is no authoritative written source of standard classifications. Complications arise because: (i) classification does not seem to correspond to physical properties of the foods; (ii) the same foods are classified differently in different cultures; (iii) a food may be classified differently by individuals within a culture; and (iv) there may be other categories or classifications of food which are superimposed on the hot–cold continuum. Grivetti (1992) summarizes data from nine publications to illustrate the variability which occurs at regional, village or even household level in Latin America. Foods labelled very hot or hot in one place may be very cold or cold in another. The most consistency is found among spices, which are nearly always hot, and fruits, which are nearly always cold.

This same author (Grivetti, 1991c) examined different published sources of yin–yang food categorization and found that of 186 foods, about three-quarters exhibited category consistency. Some 74 foods were always classified yang/hot, 12 always neutral and 60 always yin/cold. Only 22% were inconsistent, and only 13 foods were classified as both yin and yang (duck, bean sprouts, wheat, cabbage, cauliflower, green onion, mango, orange, persimmon, pineapple, honey, parsley and tea). Three foods – pork, banana and white sugar – were designated yin, neutral and yang.

Nichter offers a number of explanations for the bewildering diversity of classifications. Variation may be attributed to how individuals evaluate their physiological responses to consumption of particular foods and to inherited family traditions of classification. Individual classifications may vary over time; for example, the ability to eat a usually not-eaten food may be ascribed to a different body constitution, or to the body becoming accustomed to the food. Because foods have a number of evaluatory attributes they give mixed signals, and so may be interpreted differently by different people and at different times. Classification of food is also relationary; that is, the quality of one food is described in relation to other foods to which it may be compared or contrasted. Variance thus results according to what is being compared.

In Bangladesh, Rizvi found some indication that adherence to proscriptive rules varies with level of sophistication and economic means and with physiological state. In theory people believe attention should be paid to the hot–cold principle at all times though in everyday normal situations mothers rarely make food selections on basis of hot–cold properties. Adherence to beliefs is greater at times of stress such as illness and pregnancy and is stronger in rural villages and among non-literate urban poor. Poor mothers, being unable to meet cultural prescriptions for strength- and blood-producing foods, put more emphasis on staying away from harmful foods.

Implications for dietary practice

Grivetti (1991c) warns that conventional nutritional counselling may be ineffective among those who reject scientific values and suggests that it is necessary for nutrition educators to understand and respect lay ideologies and to adapt their own techniques accordingly. Yeung and his colleagues (1973) reported that Chinese people in Canada continued to balance hot and cold in daily meals. Western practitioners who attempt to treat Chinese clients using only scientific nutritional concepts may risk offering culturally irrelevant advice.

The consequences of not understanding non-scientific concepts is well illustrated by an example from South India. Doctors often advise the taking of milk with medicine to either enhance the patient's nutritional input or simply to associate it with this high status foodstuff. However, many patients interpreted the prescription of milk, a cooling substance, as an indication that the medicine had a heating after-effect on the body. Cases were recorded where villagers discontinued long courses of medicine because they could not afford to drink milk with the medicine. They assumed milk was a necessary part of the treatment (Nichter, 1986).

Examples presented above show that practical consequences of the various hot–cold classification systems can be, in terms of conventional nutritional wisdom, both positive and negative. There are two lessons here for the student of nutrition. The first is that a lack of understanding of traditional food classifications creates barriers to well-intentioned attempts to introduce changes in food habits. This is true not only in respect of the hot–cold ideology, but in all instances where cultural codes differ. The second lesson, perhaps more heartening to the would-be change agent, is that sound nutritional practices may, with care, be developed and reinforced within the context of existing traditional systems. Concepts of health and nutrition must be viewed in their cultural context and food habits should not be automatically labelled good or poor on the basis of modern scientific premises or rationale (Sanjur, 1982). Practices may be functionally classified as beneficial, neutral, unclassifiable or harmful. Only the latter should be subject to intervention through friendly persuasion; there is no justification for change for change's sake (Jelliffe and Bennett, 1961).

SUMMARY

The food ideology subscribed to by a given cultural group represents a collection of learned attitudes and behaviours which dictate not only what is acceptable as food but also when and how that food is to be prepared, served and eaten. Each culture tends to think of its own rules and practices as being normal, and so deviation from common practice is usually ridiculed or dismissed as being heathen or foreign – both terms of disapprobation.

Foods are categorized and classified in order to help people make sense of the world. Classifications may be based on pre-scientific understandings of inter-relationships between food and disease, on scientific nutrition knowledge of food composition, or on sociocultural uses of foods. Allopathic principles, of which the hot–cold dichotomy is the best-known expression, have a long history of informing approaches to healing and are still practised in many parts of the world today alongside scientific medicine and nutrition. Approaches to food classification by nutritional professionals have resulted in a diversity of food guides, which while claiming justification in scientific rationality nonetheless show themselves as cultural constructs with built-in biases and prejudices. The food categories used by people in their everyday lives may bear little resemblance to those of either the allopath or the scientist, but rather be based on their own cultural experience. Such differing maps of the world point up the importance of cross-cultural communication in dietary practice.

FURTHER READING

Much of the material for the section on allopathy was derived from the excellent set of four articles by Louis Grivetti (1991a,b,c, 1992), to which the reader is referred for a wealth of detail on Indian, Mediterranean, Chinese and Hispanic ideologies.

Another rich source of material, referred to in this and other chapters, is the series of essays and studies collected under the title of *Food, Society, and Culture: Aspects in South Asian Food Systems*, (eds R.S. Khare and M.S.A Rao), Carolina Academic Press, Durham.

A discussion of the evolution of food groups in the US is provided by Haughton, B., Gussow, J.D., and Dodds, J. (1987), An Historical Study of the Underlying Assumptions for United States Food Guides from 1917 Through The Basic Four Food Group Guide, *J. Nutr. Ed.*, **19**(4): 169–75.

DISCUSSION QUESTIONS

1. Compare and contrast the propositions that you are what you eat, and you eat what you are.
2. Discuss the function of food as a cultural boundary marker, using examples from your own culture or personal experience.
3. To what extent do you agree with the idea that food guides are political, as well as scientific documents?

Food ideology

4. Compare food guides from different parts of the world. To what extent do they reflect: (i) scientific consensus; (ii) customary food habits; (iii) cultural diversity; (iv) agricultural needs; and (v) environmental concerns.
5. What are the advantages and disadvantages of prescriptive food guides?
6. Are allopathic principles reconcilable with modern scientific nutrition practice?
7. What lessons can contemporary dietary practitioners learn from a study of allopathic belief systems?

CHAPTER 3

Cuisine

THE FOOD EXCHANGE

How many of us still believe that the potato originated in Ireland? That the Mediterranean, and particularly Italy, is the ancestral hearth of the tomato and its tradition of savoury sauces? That the fiery chile pepper is an ancient and enduring part of the cuisines of Indian and Southeast Asia? That the pineapple is as native to Hawaii as chocolate is to Vienna?

ELIZABETH ROZIN (1992)

Christopher Columbus never achieved his explorer's dream of sailing west to reach the East with its promise of spices and gold, but instead he unwittingly set in motion the greatest food exchange of all time. Indeed, Columbus's voyages made possible a gastronomic treasury and a nutritional status never before dreamed of (Goldblith, 1992). In the closing years of the 18th century the food plants grown in what would soon become known as the Old and the New World were almost completely different. No one crop was a significant source of food for both 'worlds'. But the advent of the European voyages of discovery was to change all that as a multitude of new foods made their way to the Old World, where they were adopted, adapted and in many cases reintroduced to America by new generations of settlers and immigrants. Some 400 years later fully one third of all plant crops used to feed humans and animals are of New World origin (Crosby, 1972). From the New World came maize, beans, peanuts, potato, sweet potato, manioc (cassava), squashes, pumpkin, papaya, guava, avocado, pineapple, tomato, chile pepper and cocoa. Together, these made the single most valuable addition to food-producing plants of the Old World since the beginning of agriculture. (Crosby, 1972). From the Old World to the New came bananas, sugar and coffee.

The Columbian exchange had a profound impact not only in Europe but in countries around the globe. The three most important new foods for Europe were the potato, maize and beans while cassava and sweet potatoes had a major impact on other continents. For example, only about 8% of human food crops had their origins in Africa. Today, American foods – maize, cassava, peanuts, squash, pumpkins and sweet potatoes – predominate in Eastern and Central Africa and are secondary crops in other parts of the continent. Lima beans, pumpkins and squash are found throughout India, which is also the world's leading producer of peanuts. The chilli pepper, unknown in 17th century India, is now an ubiquitous and indispensable ingredient in Indian meals.

Whereas the introduction of New World plants allowed farmers to utilize previously marginal land, so Old World plants and animals were vital to the growing population of American colonists. In each case, the food exchange led to rapid increases in population. While this is generally accepted to be the case for Europe, it also holds for Africa and India, where Crosby rates the importance of the spread of food crops in stimulating population growth in the 19th century above that of either medical advances, infrastructure development or political stability.

Crosby also points out that in the New World, now, there are thousands upon thousands of acres where coffee, bananas, wheat, barley and rye now occupy the land formerly grazed by native animal species. Ironically, despite the global dispersal of major food crops and their important impact on world populations, the Columbian exchange has left us with not a richer but a poorer gene pool, causing the extinction of more species of life in the last 400 years than the usual processes of evolution might kill off in a million. Nevertheless, patterns of food availability and usage stimulated by the Columbian food exchange shaped subsequent developments in global cuisines, to which we now turn.

CUISINE

> A fine sauce will make even an elephant or a grandfather palatable.
>
> *De La Reynière (1968)*

Cuisine is a term commonly used to denote a style of cooking with distinctive foods, preparation methods and techniques of eating. A national cuisine is what is, or what is thought of as, the normal or typical food of a particular country; precisely because it is 'normal' it is not thought of as an expression of individuality, but rather as an aspect of group identity. Thus when someone refers to French cuisine, or Italian cuisine; to Cantonese or Szechuan cuisine, we have an immediate idea of what kinds of foods and dishes are being described. Sometimes though, our ideas of foreign cuisines can be quite misleading, formed, as they often are, from cook books, travelogues and local restaurant interpretations of classic dishes. Stereotypes are thus created and perpetuated and we may be quite surprised on actually visiting, say Italy, to discover that not everyone eats pizza and spaghetti all the time.

Often it is difficult to define a native cuisine; what, for example, is Canadian food? As in the United States, so in Canada cuisine has been influenced not only by available native plants and techniques but also by the many cultural groups who have immigrated to the New World over the past 300 years. Practices which are now considered to be the epitome of American ways were in fact introduced by settlers from other lands. As American as apple pie? – the apple pie was bought from England; barbecued steaks? – a technique introduced by Spaniards who in turn learnt it from Caribbean natives. North American cuisine is indeed cosmopolitan; there is a willingness to borrow from other cultures that results in a tendency toward easy acceptance of new products and techniques. Most large cities offer a wide variety of ethnic restaurants, making it easy for urban dwellers to sample a dozen exotic cuisines with no more effort than a short car drive. Both the genuine ethnic dish and Americanized versions thereof are readily available, so when someone suggests 'let's eat out', the reply is: 'do you fancy Italian, Greek or Chinese – or Vietnamese or Indian or Japanese?'. Probably the single major distinguishing feature of the North American diet is the emphasis placed on meat. In summer, the air of parks and gardens is filled with the smell of large slabs of meat being ritualistically barbecued, while for those with less ambition there are the ubiquitous steak houses and the burger joints offering the reassurance of a totally familiar product. One fast food chain is currently offering the 'All Canadian Meal', consisting of a burger, french fries and soft drink.

Farb and Armelagos (1980) suggest that cuisine consists of four components: foods chosen for use, preparation methods, flavour principles and rules governing meal behaviour. To these may be added meal patterns and structures. Flavour principles are discussed in Chapter 9; the other components are considered at more length below.

FOODS CHOSEN FOR USE

In a sense, the whole of this book is devoted to the question of what foods are chosen for use by different cultural groups. Considered here are those foods which assume central importance in the diet by virtue of being staple crops, and which constitute the bulk of what is eaten. Heiser (1990) provides a detailed account of the origins and importance of the world's major staples. Because of their dietary pre-eminence such foods may come to have special ceremonial or supernatural properties associated with them. They are sometimes called 'cultural superfoods', and the word for the important staple may come to stand for food in general. It may also take on extensive symbolic significance. Thus the Christian Lord's prayer asks: 'Give us this day our daily bread'; bread is referred to as 'the staff of life'; 'bread' is used as a slang term for money – the basic means of subsistence in our Northern and Western societies.

Balfet (1976) explores the central role of bread in some Mediterranean cultures. It may be made with herbs, seeds and seasonings; eggs, cheeses, fat or bits of meat may be mixed with the dough, as in pizza. It is frequently served as a sandwich. Bread is never thrown away but given great respect, while the leaven is regarded as having hidden power. In Turkey, if a piece of bread falls to the floor or is found in the street, it is picked up and kissed before being put back on the plate or in the rubbish bin so it won't be trampled on (Schlabach, 1991). Sorghum and millet, the chief cereals of Yemen are mixed in a bread which is an indispensable part of a meal (Bornstein-Johanssen, 1976). Bread is used as a utensil to scoop up other foods. The tortilla of Latin America and the chapatti of India are flatbreads fulfilling a similar function. The breadfruit, a native plant of Tahiti is used as a bread throughout the West Indies.

> No civilization worthy of the name has ever been founded on any agricultural basis other than the cereals. The ancient cultures of Babylonia and Egypt, of Rome and Greece, and later those of north- ern and western Europe, were all based on the growing of wheat, barley, rye and oats. Those of India, China and Japan had rice for their basic crop. The pre-Columbian peoples of America – Inca, Maya and Aztec – looked to corn for their daily bread.
>
> *Mangelsdorf (1978)*

Wheat is the world's most cultivated plant. It was probably the earliest cereal to be cultivated and its domestication, says Mangelsdorf, laid the foundations of Western civilization. Wheat cultures predominate in Europe, North America, Northern Africa and Russia and are usually asso- ciated with a relatively diverse and abundant food supply. Rice cultures are found in South Asia and West Africa. Hanks (1972) describes the Rice Goddess who is central to the lives of Thai villagers; in times past when people were virtuous, rice alone sufficed to nourish them – an idea perpetuated in a fashion by modern Zen macrobiotic practices. Thais commonly eat rice at each meal and may issue an invitation to eat by asking guests if they would like to eat rice. To smash the rice pot is to destroy one's livelihood. Rice cultures have higher prevalences of the deficiency disease of Beri-Beri, due to low thiamine intakes associated with polished rice consumption.

Maize cultures are found in Latin America and parts of South America. For the native Indian peoples of much of the American continents, maize was a true cultural superfood. Dependence on maize as a staple is associ- ated with a deficiency of nicotinic acid (niacin) leading to the disease of pellagra. The African Bemba give central place to millet, which forms the bulk of their diet. Meals consist of heavy lumpy millet porridge, known as nbwali, served with a relish of vegetables and, rarely, scraps of meat or fish. Nbwali is akin to 'bread', in that it represents life and health: the word recurs in proverbs, folk tales, puns, jokes, songs and riddles, and is used extensively in rituals such as marriage ceremonies, initiation rites, political actions, kinship relations; Nbwali is a central theme in cultural life as well as being the main source of sustenance (Williams, 1973).

Millet–sorghum is the staple crop in sub-Saharan Africa and in parts of India and China, while in Central Africa, cassava (manioc) dominates. Although cassava is tolerant of poor soils and drought and is the highest yielding of tropical crops, it is nevertheless associated with endemic malnutrition because of its poor nutritional value. Root crops then, as well as cereals, can become cultural superfoods, as is illustrated in the following account of the historical ascendancy of the potato.

The potato comes to Europe

The potato is one of the crops grown in greatest quantities around the world, and has a central role in meals in Western Europe. Originating in Peru as early as 500 BC, it gained acceptance only slowly in other parts of the world. In Peru it was an important nutritional food for it thrived in poor land and at elevations where few other cultivated plants would grow. It also had an important symbolic value; the potato motif is common in Peruvian pottery samples, where it often takes an anthropomorphic design (Salaman, 1985). Moreover, the potato designs are sometimes mutilated which, suggests Salaman, represents an outpouring of blood as in a sacrifice; blood was often poured over seed potatoes to ensure fertility of the crop, and bowls of potato meal were buried with the dead.

The word potato was derived from 'batata', a native American name for the sweet potato. A number of new root crops were appearing in Europe in the 16th century and confusion arose over which was which. Introduced by the Spaniards into Europe about 1570, the potato was at first viewed with fear and scepticism. It was recognized as a member of the Nightshade family and so became identified with its poisonous cousins; some even thought it to cause leprosy. The Scots rejected the potato as an unholy food as it was not mentioned in the Bible. Early potatoes were ill-adapted to the long days of European summers and it took nearly 200 years of selective cultivation before potatoes became established as a major crop.

In Ireland, due to prevailing climatic conditions and because it fitted into existing cooking patterns, the potato was quickly accepted relatively early on. It helped the Irish peasants to survive hardships inflicted by war and strife and soon became the basic food of most of the population. The potato has been held responsible for the massive population increase in 18th century Ireland for it provided 'a maximum of sustenance with a minimum of labour' (Salaman, 1985). With a typical diet of 10 to 12 pounds of potatoes per head per day, the population increased from about 3.2 million in 1754 to 8.2 million by 1845. The Irish became so dependent on this new cultural superfood that the failure of the crop resulted in widespread famines in the mid-19th century. Because they wouldn't eat fish unless they could get potato to go with it, and because they rejected corn maize as being inedible for humans (it was called 'Peel's brimstone', after the Prime Minister of England), the Irish people suffered a famine which resulted in a halving of the population in a matter of 20 years. Desperation forced many families to emigrate to the New World. It is estimated that one-and-a-half million people died, while a further million left the country bound mainly for North America. Heiser (1990) comments that it is ironic that a New World crop – maize – was rejected as a means of sustenance, when a previously introduced New World crop failed.

Acceptance of the potato spread across Europe, generally from west to east, in response to a combination of devastating famines and subsequent deliberate government policy to promote the crop. One result was massive population increases consequent on raised nutritional standards. In comparison with its German, Italian and Belgian neighbours France was laggardly in its adoption of the potato. Early attempts to popularize it had been unsuccessful, its promoters being scorned as purveyors of pig food. In 1779 Parmentier, a pharmacist and long-time potato advocate, won a competition on the theme of plants that can replace cereals in time of famine. In 1785 he presented a bouquet of purple potato flowers to Louis XVI, insisting that from then on famine would be impossible. Potatoes were served at the French royal table and Marie Antoinette wore potato flowers in her corsage. The King also had a field of potatoes planted and heavily guarded which, of course, aroused the interest of the peasantry. When the crop matured the royal guard was withdrawn – and all of the potatoes disappeared overnight. General acceptance of the potato in France had begun.

In Russia, the introduction of the potato was at first met with open revolt; a word play equated the potato with something sexually perverse and unclean. Following the Russian famine of 1765, Catherine the Great instigated policies to promote the potato as a crop; by the mid-19th century it was well established and by the end of the century Russia had become one of the world's major producers of potatoes. Similar patterns of popular resistance to potatoes collapsing in the face of devastating famines were seen in Hungary.

The potato was introduced into North America in 1621, though probably didn't become established as a crop until it was bought over by Irish emigres to New Hampshire in 1719 (Heiser, 1990). Today, there are hundreds of varieties of potato bred to suit diverse conditions and needs, and potatoes are one of the four basic food crops in the world along with wheat, rice and maize.

Wild foods

In the olden days all our people had to do to get food was to gather what the Great Nature provided.

People of 'Ksan (1980)

Wild foods are those which are not deliberately cultivated or domesticated but which, nevertheless, make a significant contribution to human food consumption. Examples include grasses and tubers, fungi, insects, rodents and small mammals. Food balance sheets produced by the Food and Agricultural Organization (FAO) of the UN, suggest that about nine-tenths of the world's food supply is provided by just over 100 species. However, wild foods are not included in national food accounting systems, even though they may be of considerable local importance. Wild foods may have a significant impact on nutritional status and so it is important to take them into account when studying local nutritional systems.

Wild foods are important in all parts of the world, and are indeed central to some diets. For example, although maize is the predominant crop of Bungoma in Kenya, people consume at least 100 different species of vegetables and fruits. Similar patterns are seen throughout the world. In Northern Canada, First Nations people make extensive use of wild game, fish and berries.

Wild foods may be most obviously associated with hunters and gatherers, but they are also used in agricultural and pastoral societies. They can make significant contributions to the diet even in apparent monocultures. For example, rats, mice and locusts are common in croplands and may be eaten either as an intentional food source or as a means of pest control. Fish, snails and frogs, found in irrigated rice areas may, together with mushrooms, fruit and vegetables make up to 50% of the diet in North-East Thailand during the rainy season. Agricultural land may be managed to deliberately encourage wildlife; farmers plant particular trees on paddy irrigation dykes so as to attract lizards, rats and other potential food items (Grandstaff, 1986).

Pastoralists commonly include grains in their diets; grains which they either grow or which they buy or trade. In unfavourable circumstances these grain crops may themselves be supplemented or replaced by wild foods. In other pastoral groups wild foods are eaten only occasionally and do not represent an important dietary component. For instance, they are a merely a source of snack food for Masai herd boys and girls.

People who are displaced due to immigration or forced resettlement have to adapt to new food-getting strategies. Familiar foods may no longer be available, so there is a need to incorporate new food items into the diet. Recent settlers may be particularly reliant on wild foods while they establish themselves in a new geographical setting or ecological niche.

In many industrialized societies wild food is used by some as an adjunct to the everyday diet. A variety of animals and birds are hunted for sport and a proportion of these, at least, may be eaten. In England, game birds are hunted predominantly by the upper classes, while in Canada ducks and geese, elk and moose are pursued according to classless quota systems. Among the hunting set there is a certain prestige attached to these wild foods which is independent of their actual eating qualities. Poaching is simply the transgression of ownership boundaries or of state-imposed restrictions. Less important now than in previous times, poaching has historically been a means of supplementing the diet for rural landless poor.

Changing agricultural practices are leading to a decline in the use of wild foods. Agricultural clearance and the increased use of pesticides both contribute to a reduction in the supplementary food potential of insects. Availability of wild foods is reduced as forest land is cleared and collection sites are rendered inaccessible by development. In northern Manitoba massive hydroelectric projects in the mid-1970s resulted in the flooding of traditional native hunting and fishing grounds. In addition, mercury contamination of fish occurred, leading to a decrease in certain fish species in the diet.

Growing participation in the cash economy and exposure to commercial foods and drinks, with their high prestige value, are additional factors in the decrease in wild food consumption. As young people become more accustomed to commercial diets and Western lifestyles they begin to lose their familiarity with the diversity of wild foods available, which in turn contributes to the decreased usage of these foods. Access to wild foods in the Manitoba communities of God's River, Nelson House and South Indian Lake was found to be related to the presence of a hunter, fisher or trapper in the household (Campbell, Diamant and Macpherson, 1992). Wild food use decreased with each succeeding generation as traditional food procurement was usurped by purchase of commercial foods (Table 3.1). As a consequence of this, food preferences showed marked generational shifts away from wild food (Table 3.2).

Wild foods used

Leafy vegetables, grasses, tubers, fungi, insects, rodents, fish and small mammals are all used to supplement diets. North American Indians traditionally used hundreds of wild plants in their diets including stinging nettle, common purslane, milkweed, clover, pond-lily, dandelions and fiddleheads. For example, the brown spikes of cattails, growing in ponds and marshes could be eaten like corn on the cob. African cooks use wild leafy vegetables such as Amaranthus, or Red Root, to add to soups and sauces. In Zaire the Red Root leaves are pounded, using a mortar and pestle, and added to palm oil sauces. In Papua New Guinea, a section of bamboo tube may be stuffed with fresh greens and cooked over the fire.

Table 3.1 The declining use of wild foods in a Canadian aboriginal population

Older adults (56 years)	Women (25–45 years)	Women (16–25 years)	Children (1–4 years)
	Loon	Loon	Loon
	Gull eggs	Gull eggs	Gull eggs
	Brook trout	Brook trout	Brook trout
	Moose liver	Moose liver	Moose liver
	Moose kidney	Moose kidney	Moose kidney
	Lake trout	Lake trout	Lake trout
	Redsucker	Redsucker	Redsucker
	Fish liver	Fish liver	Fish liver
		Fish eggs	Moose heart
		Muskrat	Muskrat
		Lynx	Lynx
		Moose tongue	Moose tongue
			Caribou
			Beaver
			Partridge
			Smoked meat
			Goose
			Pickerel
			Beef liver
			Other store-bought fish

*The Table shows generational differences in the types of food never eaten by 50% or more of respondents in each age group in Nelson House, Manitoba.
Adapted from Campbell, M.L., Diamant, R.F. and Macpherson, B.D. (1992) *Dietary Survey of preschool children, women of child-bearing age and older adults in God's River, Nelson House and South Indian Lake*, Medical Services Branch, Health and Welfare Canada, Ottawa.

Over 13 000 insects have been classified as edible. Termites are an important fat and protein supplement across southern Africa. Locust or cricket swarms also provide important additions to local diets. One creative method of collecting termites is to saturate the termite mounds with water and then bang on drums to simulate thunder, causing the termites to leave the nest. Another method involves placing buckets beneath street lamps after a rain. The termites are attracted to the street lights and upon landing discard their wings and fall into the waiting buckets!

Fish were and are very important for the Gitksan Indians of Northern British Columbia. Fish was served at every meal, salmon, trout and mountain whitefish being preferred. Every part of the fish was eaten except for

Table 3.2 Changing food preferences in a Canadian aboriginal population

Elders	Women (25–45 years)	Women (16–25 years)	Children (1–4 years)
Moose	Bannock	Pork chops	Bacon
Pickerel	Moose	Bacon	Bologna
Strawberries	Duck	Raspberries	Chicken
Raspberries	Jackfish	Eggs	Hamburger
Blueberries	Pork chops	Potatoes	Wieners
Smoked fish	Chicken	Moose	Sausage
Pork chops	Blueberries	Stewmeat	Stewmeat
Bacon	Eggs	Bread	Pork chops
Bannock	Goose	Hamburger	Moose
Goose	Strawberries	Strawberries	Macaroni
Potatoes	Stewmeat	Ham	Ham
Jackfish	Potatoes	Chicken	Potatoes
Mossberries	Hamburger	Jackfish	Jackfish
Duck	Bacon	Blueberries	Bannock

*The table shows generational differences in ranking of mean preference scores for country and store-bought foods in God's River, Manitoba, in descending order of preference score means. (For foods eaten by 50% or more of respondents). Adapted from Campbell, M.L., Diamant, R.F. and Macpherson, B.D. (1992) *Dietary Survey of preschool children, women of child-bearing age and older adults in God's River, Nelson House and South Indian Lake*, Medical Services Branch, Health and Welfare Canada, Ottawa.

the bones which were either burnt or reassembled and returned to the water so that fish could reincarnate and come again.

Rodents form an important source of food in some agricultural communities. Further, they may be heavily harvested without undermining the sustainability of the food source. In West Africa, bush meat harvesting and trade is dominated by exploitation of the African giant rat and the grasscutter rat (Ajayi, 1974). In other instances, use of such foods is more opportunistic; Taylor (1968) reported how diets changed rapidly in Kenyan agricultural areas after rat outbreaks. Rodents may even have a prestige value. In Zimbabwe, according to Wilson (1990), roasted mice fetch a high premium as a snack food at beer parties.

Use of meat from wild animals varies by ecological region and dietary custom. In West Africa bush meat is frequently consumed, especially in areas close to remaining forest, and there are extensive markets for wild meat found in West African cities. In Guatemala, armadillo, iguana and capybara are hunted, when available, to supplement diets. In Peru, over 40% of the meat is derived from four small animals. Whitetail deer is the most plentiful big game animal found in North America today, hunted for sport and subsistence, though it was the now rare buffalo that was once the mainstay of the Plains Indians. Buffalo provided meat, tools, shelter and clothing. Cut into thin strips and dried, the meat could then be crushed

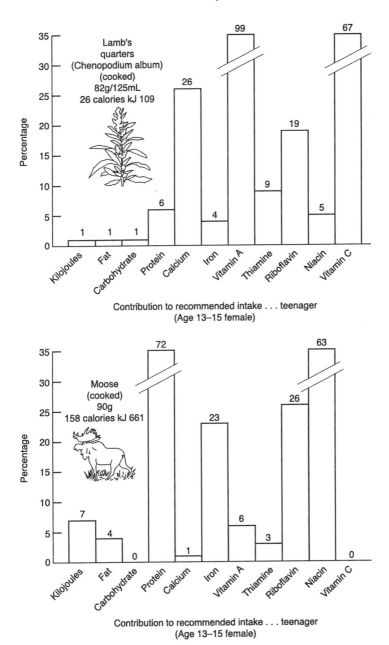

Figure 3.1 Nutritional value of Canadian wildfoods: (a) lamb; (b) moose.

Footnote: From 'Nutrient Bar Graphs – A teaching aid to learn the value of native foods, Health Canada 1984. Reproduced with permission of the Minister of Supply and Services Canada, 1994.

into powder to form pemmican. This was added to soups or mixed with various crushed berries and melted fat to form a nutritious staple.

Nutritional value

Capybara, the world's largest rodent, and iguana can have similar protein, fat and energy content as pigs, cattle and chicken. Moreover, capybara is several times more efficient at converting food to meat than is domestic cattle. Rats have a nutritional score equivalent to beef or mutton (Kyle, 1987). Ants, grubs and caterpillars have similar energy protein and fat as goose liver, pork sausage and beef liver. Beetle larvae eaten by the Tukanoa Indians of Colombia contain 24.3 g protein per 100 g, while termites contain 58.9 g per 100 g as compared with 43.4 g per 100 g for smoked river fish. While wild food eaten year round is often an important dietary component, seasonal variations in food intake from different wild sources have direct effects on nutritional status of populations. During the rainy season insects contribute 12% of the total animal protein to the diets of men and 26% to women of the Tukanoa (Dufour, 1987). Some Canadian examples of nutritional profiles of wild foods are shown in Figure 3.1.

Hunt (1992) provides recipes for a wide variety of North American wild food, including such delicacies as spicy elk meat balls, roast bear in raisin sauce, fried woodchuck and squirrel fricassee as well as many game bird and fish dishes. An intriguing recipe for buffalo is shown in Table 3.3.

Table 3.3 Tucker's stew for an army

2 large-sized buffalo	Brown gravy (lots)
2 rabbits (optional)	Salt and pepper to taste

Cut buffalo into bite-sized pieces, (this will take about 2 months, so start early). Reserve the heads and tails as you will need something to store the pieces in.

After it is all cut up, put in a large pot and add enough brown gravy to cover the meat.

Vegetables, etc. may be added at this time to taste. Cook stew over a kerosene fire about 4 weeks at 400°F. Periodically add water and stir.

This will serve about 3937 people. If more guests are expected, the two rabbits may be added, but do this only if necessary as most people do not like fine hare in their stew.

Wild foods continue to be an important component of the diet in many societies. Their nutritional value should not be underestimated, and development projects should take account of potential impacts on wild food resources.

MEAL PATTERNS

Hunger is a drive which arises periodically, and people of all cultures take at least one meal in a 24-hour period. However, patterns of meal taking vary widely and are a part of cultural learning. Thus the British typically have four 'food events' in the day, North American practice favours three daily meals, while in continental Europe, five or six 'food events' are common. There are, of course, considerable variations within the framework of general patterns and there is some evidence of a general trend away from a small number of large meals to a greater number of small meals as the norm in Northern and Western societies. Changes in family structure and in lifestyles mean that communal meals are less common and that snacks are often fitted into busy schedules as and when time allows. In India, the poor may subsist on a single daily meal, while better-off groups plan on two main meals – lunch and dinner, and two small ones – breakfast and afternoon tea. As in the West, this cycle has been blurred by modern living and working conditions.

Cultural meal patterns may develop as means to cope with acute or chronic food shortages. In some African tribes a meal is eaten only once a day. Children are taught voluntary control of the hunger drive and learn to feel hungry only at the appropriate time. In Bemba society children are permitted light snacks throughout the day, but by adolescence they are expected to adopt the adult one-meal pattern. Because of environmental conditions, the Bemba are rarely able to produce enough of their staple millet crop to last an entire year. They call the last 3 months of the year the hunger months. When millet becomes scarce the whole community slows down. Adults reduce their food intake and stop brewing millet beer; children eat only one small meal per day. Everyone curtails activity, staying in their huts and drinking large quantities of water and taking snuff to reduce their hunger (Williams, 1973).

The development of customs of fasting which make a virtue out of necessity by delaying or displacing the hunger drive is a not uncommon way of coping with food scarcities. Aids to hunger suppression are commonly employed. Coca leaves are chewed by Andean Indians in lieu of food as cocaine inhibits hunger and fatigue and also, during long arduous journeys in mountainous terrain, relieves travellers of the need to add the weight of food supplies to already large burdens. Peyote has a similar effect, as does the betel nut; hunger and thirst are inhibited and energy-requiring activity is decreased. Tobacco, coffee and tea may likewise be used to blunt appetite.

Meal patterns, including number of meals and frequency of eating, differ not only between, but also within cultural groups. The traditional English breakfast of fried bacon, sausage and eggs, followed by toast and marmalade with gallons of tea may no longer be the norm in middle-class households, but it is still offered with pride to guests at hotels and bed-

and-breakfast places and on British Rail's *Inter-City* morning trains. Elsewhere, the continental breakfast of rolls and coffee has become a firmly established alternative, partly as a result of cultural exchange, foreign travel and time consciousness and partly, perhaps, because of anxiety over dietary calories and cholesterol. Within Britain there are many regional variations in meal patterns and in preferred foods. Yorkshiremen traditionally enjoy fatty bacon, which distresses the stomachs of their more sensitive neighbours. An episode in James Herriot's memoirs of life as a vet in rural Yorkshire recalls the time when, after an early morning's job, Herriot was offered a real farm breakfast. When the bacon arrived, there was scarcely any red meat on it – a cause for admiration on behalf of the farmer but a sore trial for Herriot, who had to somehow force himself to swallow this 'delicacy'.

Even the names given to food events may vary, and the names themselves take on different meanings over time (Table 3.4). Both Western and Indian schemes classify meals by combining criteria of the time at which they are taken and quantity or type of foods eaten. Western lunch and dinner refer to size of meals more than particular time – though lunch has become associated with noon. The Indian scheme uses a generic term for all meals (bhojana or âhâra or khânâ) as it is thought to be unnecessary to specify the chief meal of the day for the whole of society (Khare, 1986). In England, the Southerner's 'dinner' is often known as 'tea' in the Midlands and North, though both terms refer to the same evening meal. (In Australia, 'tea' can be almost any refreshment break except breakfast but it usually indicates a substantial evening meal, preferably with wine.). 'Dinner' is the Northerner's mid-day meal – elsewhere known as 'lunch'; while his hearty 'tea' commonly becomes a light afternoon snack in other parts of the country. There are social class variations in meal term usage which may be more pronounced than regional differences. Whatever the meal is called, though, its structure remains remarkably consistent.

Table 3.4 The linguistic evolution of lunch

Origin:	Spanish lonja – a slice of ham
16th Century	Thick piece, hunk
1755	As much food as one's hand can hold*
18th Century	Slight repast between morning meals
19th Century	Light midday meal

*Dr. Johnson's Dictionary

Meal structure

Meals exhibit underlying structures which change little over time. Although experiments and innovations may be introduced along with new food products, the meal has to remain recognizably the same. In other words, most people have an idea of what would be acceptable as breakfast or dinner or supper, and are able to differentiate these meals from snacks. Studies of the food habits of Italian Americans in Philadelphia showed that while use of particular foods, recipes and menus varied considerably at the level of the individual, there was a consistency in meal structures and patterns at the social level, which contributed to maintaining group identity and social cohesion (Goode, Curtis and Theophano, 1984).

Douglas and Nicod (1974) conducted research into meal structures in Britain as a way of determining the likely acceptability of culinary innovations. They hypothesized that while only small reinforcing changes might be possible in the highly structured parts of food patterns, new foods and techniques could be introduced into less-structured elements of the traditional diet. Nicod actually lodged with a number of families in order to discreetly observe normal food habits. Three kinds of meals were identified; a major hot meal at about 6 p.m. on weekdays and early afternoon on weekends; a minor meal at about 9 p.m. weekdays and 5 p.m weekends; and a tertiary meal – often a biscuit and hot drink – available at different times. Breakfast was defined as a snack rather than as a meal as it did not have a consistent structure or composition. The three-meal system focused on potato and cereal; the most important meal featuring potatoes, while the minor meal included bread and possibly cakes and biscuits; the tertiary meal included biscuits.

The researchers show that the Sunday meal sequence – main, minor, tertiary – is either fitted into weekday patterns starting with the main meal at 6 p.m. or is adopted in its entirety (e.g. with the mid-day provision of cooked major meals at works canteens). They analyse the structure of the major meal, illustrating various rules of combination and order. The authors comment that the rules for structuring the first course of a major meal are absolutely strict. No deviation is allowed if the food event is to be recognized a major meal. The three courses of the major meal are structured similarly to the three meals of Sunday; that is, there is a direct structural correspondence between course 1 and the major 'potato' meal; course 2 and the minor 'cereal' meal; course 3 and the tertiary 'biscuit' meal. The role of the biscuit as a unique expression of the conclusion of a meal or meal sequence in British cuisine is emphasized.

Such a detailed analysis of meal structure (and the authors provide more insights than are recounted here) may at first seem to be mere exotica, and to be without practical implications. However, if rules for meal structures are indeed firmly adhered to then the scope for introducing new foods or for altering food behaviours is formally delimited. Nutrition educators should perhaps be aware of this when they attempt to 'improve' or modify diets. As an example, Douglas and Nicod point out that there is no place for plain fresh fruit within the meal system described and so suggestions that fresh fruit replace puddings as an economy or nutritional measure are almost inevitably doomed to failure.

In contrast to the British pattern described above, Japanese meals are not served in courses. Instead many small dishes of different types of food – hot and cold, savoury and sweet – are served, each on its own plate. At a family meal these dishes may appear on the table all at once or in random order, while more formal meals are presented according to cooking method. Traditionally, an odd number of dishes, usually either three or five, is served. Meals nearly always finish with rice, pickles and miso soup.

METHODS OF PREPARATION

'With patience, you can even cook stones'.

Hausa proverb

Methods of food preparation are diverse and many; they are related to types of food available, the state of the material culture and the cultural needs and preferences of the society. A wealth of information on methods and techniques can be found in modern cookbooks and in anthropology texts, and the topic is dwelt on but briefly here to highlight a few examples of cultural influences on, and consequences of, food preparation.

The greatest revolution in food preparation must have been the discovery of fire. Meats could be eaten raw, but cooking improved their flavour and palatability, while many vegetable foods are only edible if cooked. Early cooking methods would have included direct-heat roasting, boiling in water heated by hot stones, and the use of animal stomachs as cooking vessels. The People of 'Ksan (1980) list boiling, toasting, barbecuing, aging, smoking, sun-drying, air-drying and oven-baking as traditional food preparation methods. Red cedar boxes were used to hold water boiled by adding heated stones, while foods to be baked were wrapped in birch bark. The invention of pottery would have considerably extended options for mixing and heating foods. Topography may have placed limitations on the use of particular methods and therefore of certain foods; for example, cereals and beans are not usually popular in mountainous regions because of the inordinate amount of time required to prepare them. To bring a pan of water to the boil, of course, takes much longer in the high mountains than at sea-level, and is doubly inefficient where fuel resources are often scarce. Fuel conservation may also be achieved by cutting food into small pieces which can be cooked quickly. On the other hand, the dung fuel used in many countries of the South provides a low heat ideal for prolonged slow cooking of dishes which can be left all day while other domestic and agricultural tasks are attended to. These examples suffice to indicate that available energy has a direct impact on the types of foods which can be readily prepared and thus on cuisine.

Cultural lifestyles and occupations impose their own requirements for dishes which are 'instant', 'slow-cooking', 'oven-to-table' or easily carried. As an example of the latter, the Cornish pasty was invented as a convenient 'packaging' for meat and potatoes so that they could be eaten by miners at the pitface. Many other cultures have their own version of this packaged meal, such as Caribbean roti and East Indian samosa.

Preparation methods can add to or detract from the nutritional value of a food. It is fairly well known that prolonged boiling of vegetables leaches water-soluble vitamins into the cooking water which is often discarded with a consequent loss of valuable nutrients. The addition of baking soda to green vegetables to keep them brightly coloured also reduces nutritional value. Dripping from roasted meats contain nutrients, lost unless the drippings form the basis of a gravy. On the other hand some methods of preparation actually enhance nutritional value. Pellagra is a disease endemic to many maize-eating societies. For many years, before the elucidation of vitamin deficiency theories, it was held to be an infectious disease so widespread was its occurrence. Even with discovery of a link between niacin deficiency and the symptoms of pellagra some puzzling anomalies remained. Pellagra was observed in some groups who had higher average intakes of niacin than other groups who were pellagra-free. Even after the quantity of tryptophan in the diet had been taken into account (tryptophan is an amino acid which can under certain conditions be converted to niacin) the differences in disease prevalence persisted. The solution to the puzzle lay in the discovery that niacin occurs in a bound form in maize and thus its actual biological availability is low. The technique of soaking maize in lime water to soften it before using it in baking has the effect of freeing niacin from its bound form and making it available. This cultural practice helps then to explain why some maize eaters do not suffer from pellagra. A further example of nutritional enhancement is found among the Pima Indians of Arizona, where three methods of preparation all have the effect of increasing calcium levels in food. They are, roasting of food in contact with coals or ashes; grinding of food with stone grinding implements; and cooking of corn in a Mesquite ash solution. In the first two instances iron levels are also raised. When assessing the nutritional adequacy of a diet it is important to consider the potential effects of nutrient losses or additions during food preparation in order to arrive at accurate conclusions.

The culinary triangle

Not only have foods themselves been categorized in a variety of ways which reflect how we think about them, but methods of food preparation too have been analysed with a view to understanding both social structure and human thought processes. Food preparation as a cultural phenomenon has been explored in immense detail by Claude Levi-Strauss, a leading exponent of structuralism. According to Levi-Strauss the way in which we perceive relationships in nature leads us to generate cultural products which incorporate the same kind of relationships. He claims that cultural elements have a common inner structure that reflects the common structure of human thought, and that by searching for underlying universals of human culture we can learn about human nature. Just as every human society has a language there is no society which does not process at least some of its food by cooking. 'Communication and food are the things that one lives by', says a Somali proverb. Cooking is a universal means by which nature is transformed into culture, and categories of cooking are therefore eminently appropriate as symbols of social organization and differentiation (Leach, 1970).

Although the kinds of foods available to different human sub-groups varies considerably, every society breaks up those foods which are available into a number of categories, each of which is treated in a different way. Levi-Strauss (1969) claims that cross-culturally these categories are remarkably alike, and he identifies them as raw, cooked and rotted. Cooked food is raw food which has been transformed by cultural means, whereas rotted food is fresh raw food which has been transformed by natural means. The principal modes of cooking food – roasting, boiling and smoking – also form a structured set, but one which is in opposition to the first. Levi-Strauss constructed a culinary triangle in which natural versus cultural and prepared versus unprepared properties of food are linked (Figure 3.2).

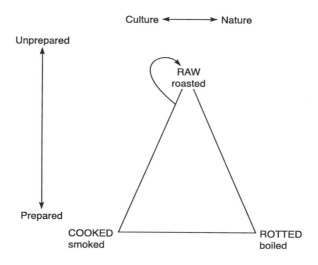

Figure 3.2 The culinary triangle.

Roasted food is directly exposed to fire without the intervention of cultural apparatus and therefore belongs to nature and also to the unprepared category; boiled food must be cooked in vessels made by humans and is therefore in the cultural and the prepared category; smoked foods are prepared with the mediation of air but without cultural apparatus and thus belong to the natural and prepared categories. Roasted food has an affinity with raw as it is never uniformly cooked; boiled food may be linked with rotted, as both processes – natural and cultural – reduce food to a decomposed state; ('potpourri' means rotted pot); and smoked can be associated with cooked food. Levi-Strauss elaborates on this simple triangle, incorporating other methods of food preparation such as grilling and frying in a more complex diagram. He believes that the system which emerges can be applied to other aspects of society and thus that food preparation is a kind of language which tells us something about societal structure. Indeed, the categories of food as indicated in the culinary triangle are widely accorded very different levels of social prestige. Roasted food is special; it is of high status; it is for men. Boiled food is everyday; it is suitable for children and invalids. It is significant that people in different cultures sort out their foodstuffs in very similar ways and apply similar status distinctions. Levi-Strauss has even claimed that the high status attached to roasted food is a universal cultural characteristic. If this is true, then by studying the use of roasted food in a society – who prepares it, who eats it, when and where it is eaten – we can not only learn a lot about the social structure of that particular human group, but also about the way in which people think.

Levi-Strauss's theories have been heavily criticized because of his use of selective and often exotic examples with which to prove his point, which arouses suspicions that he has simply chosen those particular examples which will fit into his pre-arranged matrix while ignoring those that are problematical (Leach, 1970). He has also been accused of making sweeping generalizations which are not always supported by empirical evidence. Despite such criticisms, it is true that Levi-Strauss has accumulated much evidence for the existence of common structural principles underlying the way in which foods and food preparation methods are categorized.

RECIPE REPERTOIRES

All recipes are built on the belief that somewhere at the beginning of the chain there is a cook who does not use them – an absent mother-cook who once laid her hands on the body of the world for us and worked it into food. The promise of every cookbook is that it offers a way back into her lap.

Thorne (1990)

While nutritionists have focused on the value of food on the plate they have often neglected to address the question of how it got there. Domestic food consumption begins with what is bought; what is bought and what is served are in turn circumscribed by the ability to prepare the food. It seems unlikely that consumers will buy foods which they do not know how to prepare or that they will attempt to prepare dishes which make undue demands on their cookery skills.

Recipes are an everyday phenomenon in industrial society but they do not exist, at least in written form, in pre-literate societies or indeed in many contemporary developing countries. In this case there may be mental equivalents to the written list, used routinely and derived from observation and experience or passed on from generation to generation. The very idea of writing down the instructions for making a simple dish may seem quite strange. Thus in Botswana, for example, recipes are seldom recorded, while in rural Bangladesh experience and experimentation replace strict use of recipes.

The word 'recipe' is derived from the Latin verb 'to take' and replaces the older term, 'receipt'. Originally it referred to medical prescriptions but is now used more generally to describe a formula for action – especially one which sets out details for the preparation of food. Popular wisdom defines a recipe as a list of ingredients and instructions for combining them to produce a dish, though there is obviously more to it than that. As well as providing rules for food preparation recipes encode cultural knowledge and transmit it inter-generationally.

However, even if we start with the idea that a recipe is simply a tool which can be used to 'manufacture' a product (a dish or a meal) the practical implications for nutrition education are obvious. The range of tools at an individual's disposal governs the range of possible meals which can be produced. When faced with the challenge of changing their food habits, whether for health or social purposes, food preparers must look for suitable new tools. If these are not available or if they cannot successfully be deployed then change will be more difficult. As a corollary to this the nutrition educator may find that the provision of new tools (recipes) is a vehicle for introducing nutritionally desirable changes.

The sense of this proposition has theoretical and pragmatic support. Health belief models suggest that in order to put new ideas into practice there must be suitable provision for action, or facilitating factors which support 'doing'. Pragmatically, food manufacturers and supermarkets have for a long time used recipe leaflets as a marketing tool. New products are supported with instructions as to how to prepare attractive and tasty meals. To a certain extent this has happened in health promotion too, with healthful recipes being part of the resource backup for nutrition interventions. One Canadian initiative, 'The Light Gourmet' combines a video series featuring famous guest chefs with printed recipes endorsed by the Heart and Stroke Foundation of Canada and the Canadian Cancer Society.

Cookery books were among the earliest printed books in Europe. The first one in English, concerned with the practices and needs of the nobility, was *This is the Boke of Cokery*; it was not until a century later, in 1615, that the middle class gentlewoman was addressed in Markham's *The English Hus-Wife*. At first, cookery books included medical receipts and other general information, but they soon emerged as a distinct genre. Being written in vulgar tongue rather than Latin they were probably aimed at practising cooks. Nevertheless, because literacy levels were higher among the upper classes and artisans than among the peasants, cookery practices, informed by this new written means of communication, changed more rapidly in the courts and cities than in the countryside (Mennell, 1985). The advent of written collections of recipes had both conservative and progressive effects. On the one hand, they replaced apprenticeships and personal relationships as the only means of passing on skills and knowledge. By making possible the preparation of a variety of dishes far beyond the conception of one individual recipe books allowed for the transcending of regional and cultural food boundaries. In so doing they can be seen as having had a democratising and empowering influence; private knowledge was made public and cooks could test, adapt and improve on one another's creations. Mennel comments that in 18th century France recipes and styles of eating had become matters of high fashion. Recipe books showed how basic peasant fare could be elaborated into dishes fit for the court, while aristocratic dishes were popularized for the less wealthy. On the other hand, committing recipes to print made them more prescriptive. The act of writing them down rendered them more permanent and less open to change; a label or title was attached, ingredients were standardized and, later, precise quantities were specified, all of which reduced individual idiosyncrasy and exerted pressures toward conformity and conservatism (Mennel, 1985). In John Thorne's view the recipe collection – the cookbook – is the original kitchen machine. It helped to reduce the richness of lived experience into a succession of mechanical steps. As more and more sophisticated technologies such as food processors and microwave ovens came into common use the depersonalization of cooking was exacerbated by reducing the need for skills as well as for personal knowledge. Viewed in this way, exclusive use of recipe cooking may lead to the loss of cuisine as a complex amalgam of tradition, prejudice, shared skills and available ingredients (Thorne, 1990). Indeed, recipes can only provide a guide to how foods are prepared; they cannot 'capture the graceful art of chopping vegetables or the rhythmic kneading of bread dough. Neither can they offer the friendships that develop while learning to cook from another person.' (Schlabach, 1991). Indigenous recipes, as opposed to those developed in commercial test kitchens, can tell stories, illuminating the culture of their place of origin and reflecting the way of life and material resources of their users.

It is by no means clear then that the recipe is merely a tool. It also undoubtedly has symbolic values, one of which is to connote power and control; hence the significance of secret recipes and family recipes passed from generation to generation. Refusing to disclose the recipe of an admired dish enhances the cook's status as the possessor of a special talent or power, while sharing recipes is a social act akin to sharing the actual food. Endless speculation about the ingredients in Coca-Cola soft drink or Colonel Sander's chicken coating endows these products with a certain mystique and adds to their enduring attraction. Despite the plethora of recipes readily available in a thousand magazines and books there is still a certain social cache to be the one who discovers a particular recipe, to the extent that that person may actually assume or be awarded ownership of it by peers. Thus we have 'Corinne's Cranberry Streuselkuchen', in popular demand at festive occasions, but only ever made by Corinne.

Recipes are also examples of written codified rules which require of their users both an ability and a willingness to follow the rules. This presupposes skills of literacy and numeracy and the ability to follow sequential instructions. In the absence of such skills recipes may actually have a de-skilling effect in that inability to follow the rules may debar an individual from recognized achievement. If you cannot follow a recipe, you cannot cook. That this is a cultural construct is evident by the fact that quantified recipes are not used in many parts of the world. Instead, ingredients are measured in handfuls and pinches rather than in cups and tablespoons, ounces or grams; and are prepared to meet personal and local preferences rather than to produce a standard product. Ingredients may be flexible in the face of economic constraints or seasonal availability, and may change over time as a function of acculturation when people relocate. This bending of the rules does occur to a greater or lesser extent among users of written recipes and it is interesting to ask whether there are any differences in such risk taking associated with gender, age or social status.

In order to understand the meaning and usages of recipes in everyday life, as well as to assess the potential effectiveness of the recipe as a tool for change, it is necessary to understand how recipes are conceptualized by food preparers. Although the sale of magazines and cookery books is enormous, common observation seems to suggest that most people have a fairly limited range of dishes which they prepare on a regular basis. This might be termed their 'recipe repertoire'. How such repertoires are acquired, expanded and drawn upon has significance for food habits.

Techniques of eating

Before the introduction of the fork as a utensil, foods were commonly scooped up in breads or by fingers alone. Breads such as pittas in Europe, chapattis and pooris in India and tortilla in Mexico are still used almost as utensils. Carol Rose, contributing to a cross-cultural cookbook, describes the lunch practices of a silk group cooperative in NaLao in north-east Thailand. Each member contributes to the common spread – baskets of steamed sticky rice, bowls of spicy fish sauce, steamed greens, banana flowers, boiled bamboo shoots, squash and papaya. Using no utensils, they reach their fingers into the serving dishes, forming balls of sticky rice and dipping it into the sauces (Schlabach, 1991). In the US, finger foods are associated with informal occasions and are not a normal part of regular meals; in other societies, the use of hands is essential. Farley Mowat (1965) describes his first meal with Canadian Inuit:

> The tray was magnificent, but its contents were even more impressive. Half a dozen parboiled legs of deer were spread out in a thick gravy which seemed to be composed of equal parts of fat and deer hairs. Bobbing about in the debris were a dozen tongues and, like a cage holding the lesser cuts of meat, there was an entire boiled rib basket of a deer.... The etiquette of the situation eluded me. I took my sheath knife and cautiously sawed off a good sized chunk of leg meat, scraped the encrustation of hairs from it, and cuddled it in my lap since there was nothing else that could serve as a plate.

> Now Franz and the three Ihalmiut men tusked in – I use that word advisedly – and Ohot seized an entire leg. Sucking the gravy from it with appreciative lips, he sank his teeth into the tough muscle while with his left hand he held the joint away from his face, and with his right hand made a quick slash at the meat with his knife.... Hekwaw seemed to prefer the soup. He dipped his cupped hands in it and then sucked up the greasy fluid with gusty relish, taking time out now and again to chew at a deer's tongue which he dropped back into the soup to keep warm between bites.

This description might well have been applied to mealtimes in Medieval Europe. Before the introduction of eating utensils table manners were what would today be considered disgusting. Food was eaten from common dishes, plucked out of sauces by unwashed hands and discarded on the floor or even back into the pot. Soups would be slurped from the bowl, and drinks swigged from communal cups passed freely around. Elias (1978) presents some instructive quotations from 13th century treatises which show early attempts to enforce what we might regard as minimally polite table manners.

From the nature of the injunctions it was obviously common practice to spit out food, put it back in the dish, and to offer to others foods which had already been bitten into. At first, such rules of etiquette as those mentioned above were directed at courtly practice; as the bourgeoisie attempted to imitate or prepare for entry into the court they too adopted the new rules of behaviour, in turn influencing provincial practices. Thus the new customs were disseminated from the upper class downwards, and were subsequently adopted by 'civilized' society as a whole. By the 19th century, the whole movement which had generated manners had been forgotten, and proper behaviour at table was taken for granted; what had so recently gone before was now labelled barbaric. Since then there have been few substantial changes in etiquette and techniques of eating remain basically unchanged.

The manner in which meals are served has changed considerably from the Middle Ages to modern times, and this itself has affected eating techniques. For example, it was common in Medieval upper class households to have the whole dead animal, or substantial parts of it, brought to the table for carving. The privilege of carving and distributing the meat was a particular honour and the ability to carve was thus an indispensable accomplishment of a man of breeding. During the 17th century this practice started to go out of fashion, perhaps in deference to female sensibility, and it became relegated to the status of a behind-the-scenes practice to be done by servants and menials. Today, we usually try to avoid any reminders that the meat dish on our plate has anything to do with the killing of an animal, though carving the joint remains as an English tradition to be carried out on high status occasions and celebratory feasts. In this gradual removal of meat from pride of place at the table there may be implications for the future of meat-eating and vegetarianism – a theme which is taken up in Chapter 7.

The presentation of large amounts of meat at table demanded the extensive use of knives, both for carving and as the most important eating utensil. There were few restrictions on the use of knives and it was taken for granted that they were lifted to the mouth for purposes of eating. Knives were at first pointed, but were later ground down both as a safety measure and for reasons of etiquette. 'In 1669 a royal edict of Louis XIV, probably issued with a view to discourage assassination at meal-times, made it illegal for anyone to carry pointed knives, for cutlers to make them, or for inn-keepers to put them on their tables; it also commanded that any existing knives with pointed blades should have their points rounded off.' (Bailey, 1927). Although one might cut oneself when eating from a knife the element of danger in using knives has been overplayed. According to Elias (1978) it is the generalized symbolic meaning of danger which underlies the later restrictions and taboos placed on the knife. Knives are passed handle first because of the implicit and emotive threat of offering the point; we do not put knives to our mouths because that represents potential danger and would discomfort others. Consequently, the use of the knife has been gradually restricted and there is a continuing trend to use it less and less. Knives are only necessary when large pieces of food are presented on the plate. Even then, North Americans favour the use of fork only, and after cutting food as necessary, frequently lay the knife aside. Chinese food, which is pre-cut into bite-size pieces does not require the use of a knife; instead, chopsticks are an efficient technique of handling food, acting basically, as an extension of finger and thumb. Elias speculates that eventually the knife may follow the pattern set by the joint of meat, and be banished from the table altogether.

The correct use of utensils is limited and defined by a multiplicity of very precise rules the reasons for which are not self-evident. They only appear apparent to us because they have been culturally learnt and internalized. Why, for example, did civilized eating require the use of forks? It was not for hygienic reasons, as we might now suppose, but rather to spare the user the shame of being seen with soiled hands. Use of the fingers in eating led to a number of other unavoidable piggish manners which were deemed to be disagreeable and offensive. Forks appeared in Italy about 1600 CE (Common Era) and were at first derided as being silly and effete. They were not generally used in England until the mid-18th century. From then on, table utensils continued to become more elaborate and differentiated; and instead of communal implements everyone had his or her own set of utensils each with its specific use.

Customs form and evolve gradually in response to the structure of society and to changes in human relationships. Thus Medieval advice on etiquette was aimed at the upper class so that they would know how to behave at court, and not because of any intrinsic value attached to the new behaviours themselves. Adopting the new manners was a mark of 'civilite'; as the practices spread throughout society they no longer served as distinguishing marks of the elite and so further refinements had to be made in order to maintain a social separation. As the concept of civilite pervaded society as a whole, it was absorbed into normal practice and ceased to be commented on. We tend to assume that manners were refined and utensils introduced for reasons of hygiene, whereas the real motivation stemmed from the idea that civilized people behaved in certain ways.

SUMMARY

Cuisine is a distinctive cultural phenomenon. Featured foods depend on the dominant domesticated staples, resources gathered or hunted from the wild and, increasingly, availability of manufactured products. These foods are treated to a variety of preparation methods using written or oral rules to transform them, and are presented at culturally sanctioned times of day to be eaten in ways deemed socially acceptable. The traveller in a foreign land has many hazards to negotiate in adjusting to new eating behaviours, as does the immigrant in a newly adopted country. The foods on offer may be substantially different from normal fare, while the etiquette of eating may prove to be elusive and challenging.

Cultural cuisine is maintained through continuity in a set of culture-specific food practices which includes the frequent use of a basic set of foods, characteristic flavourings and preparation methods in a framework of social rules governing everyday and celebratory meal structures and patterns. Shared food habits provide a sense of belonging; they are an affirmation of cultural identity and as such are not easily given up. The fact that it is hard to retain a commitment to cultural relativism; hard to accept that one's own practices are simply the product of one codified system among many, indicates the great importance we attach to our food habits. Our unwillingness to accept just anything as food, betrays the notion that food is consumed for nourishment of the body alone. Food also nourishes the heart, mind and soul.

FURTHER READING

For a detailed account of the impact of Columbus' voyages, which goes beyond food, see Crosby (1972). For comprehensive accounts of the history and role of food plants, Simmonds' (1976) edited book provides concise overviews of individual foods, while Heiser (1990) presents a contextual treatment which is highly recommended. Root (1980) and Masefield *et al.* (1969) are also excellent sources.

Accounts of the cuisines of over 100 ethnic groups in Canada are included in Barer-Stein's comprehensive study. Her book also includes valuable background information on topics such as special occasions and home life (Barer-Stein, 1979).

The major reference source for the wild foods section was *The Hidden Harvest: Wild Foods and Agricultural Systems. A literature review and annotated bibliography*, edited by Scoones, Melnyk and Pretty and published jointly by the World Wide Fund for Nature, the Swedish International Development Agency and the International Institute for Environment and Development. Over 900 annotated citations are included, providing a wealth of information to which the interested reader is referred.

Hunt's comprehensive book on wild foods in contemporary North America contains over 300 recipes plus information on nutritional contributions of selected wild foods, and useful cooking tips such as 'To remove the gamey taste from a beaver, add a tablespoon of coffee to the water when parboiling' and 'When cooking the snapping turtle; after removing the head, be very careful not to touch the head for at least 24 hours, as the nerves remain alive for at least that amount of time.' Many of the recipes are derived from a research project conducted by the Lovesick Lake

Native Women's Association in Ontario. Hunt, D. (ed.) (1992), *Native Indian Wild Game, Fish and Wild Foods Cookbook*, Fox Chapel Publishing, Lancaster, Pennsylvania.

Two books by Margaret Visser explore the everyday anthropology of eating. *Much Depends on Dinner*, (McClelland and Stewart, Toronto 1986) focuses on foods selected for an everyday meal, while *The Rituals of Dinner* (HarperCollins, Toronto, 1991) is a wide-ranging examination of the origins, evolution, and meaning of table manners in historical and contemporary societies.

Stephen Mennel (*All Manners of Food*, Blackwell Science, Oxford, 1985) provides a fascinating social history of the development of cookery in England and France, over the past four centuries.

DISCUSSION QUESTIONS

1. Compare the effects of the modern multinational food system with those of the Columbian food exchange in the area of food availability.
2. Identify and discuss the uses of the contemporary cultural superfoods in your country or region.
3. Discuss the advantages and disadvantages of encouraging the use of wild foods in modern industrial societies.
4. Contrast the empowering and de-skilling attributes of recipes. Are these culture-specific?
5. Are recipes a conservative or innovative force in today's world?
6. Suggest some possible research approaches to further investigating the concept of recipe repertoires and their practical implications.
7. Investigate regional and local variations in meal names in your own, or a selected geographical area.

CHAPTER 4

Social functions of food

While it is true that food and the act of eating have innumerable non-biological associations and meanings, nowhere is this more evident than in the common everyday experiences of social interaction. For food is a vehicle for expressing friendship, for smoothing social intercourse, for showing concern. It is also ridden with status symbolism and is manipulated, subtly or blatantly, to demonstrate differences in social standing. There might almost be a dictum which says where two or more people gather together then let there be food and drink. Rituals and celebrations are usually centred around food; sometimes the type of food served can define the event, as with the Thanksgiving turkey or the Christmas pudding. The major transitional crises of life, the rites of passage, are marked in almost all societies by ritual or ceremonial distribution and consumption of food. Cohen (1968) hypothesizes that these important life events signify changes in socioeconomic relationships and responsibilities; as food usages commonly symbolize social relationships changes in the latter are noted symbolically by displays, exchanges and consumption of foods.

Food is distributed and shared according to complex rules and customs which reflect social values and structures. Cohen identifies four common patterns. Recurrent exchange and sharing is a feature of societies where community solidarity is maximal. Kin groups are highly integrated, families live in close physical proximity, and there is little change in community membership. Under these conditions there is an almost constant flow of food between groups. Among the Wamirans of Papua New Guinea, pigs are controlled and exchanged by men; they are symbols of female sexuality. 'Unable to master women, men master pigs which serve as tangible, manipulable and composite symbols of the unharnessable characteristics of women' (Kahn, 1986). Pigs and women are seen as economic and social extensions of individual men, and exchanges of both are valuable in linking men and maintaining male relationships; men exchange pigs and pork with the same people with whom they exchange women for marriage. Piglet exchanges are ways of maintaining links between affines, forcing men to engage in repetitive and reciprocal exchange and reinforcing the connection between a married woman and her own lineage members.

Mutual assistance and sharing in times of need is characteristic of a second type of social structure. Although kinship ties are still strong there is greater physical mobility and change in community membership. Communal sharing of a hunter's kill, and willingness to help in times of economic difficulties would be typical of this type of structure. Narrowed and reluctant sharing, Cohen's third type, is characterized by reluctant and grudging rendering of assistance between social units. It is associated with a fragmented social system in which the isolated nuclear family is the predominant social form. Food is served to the immediate family only, and this serves to define the boundaries of the family and to symbolize its separateness from other nuclear families. Physical and social distance is great, and there are rarely any functioning kin groups outside the immediate family. Although ideals of generosity and mutual assistance in times of need are articulated, in practice they are severely restricted in quality and quantity and to a limited group, usually based on kinship. Finally, non-sharing is characteristic of societies in which there are no stable social groupings and where the accumulation of individual wealth and power is paramount. Cohen comments that this is an uncommon social form, citing the Alorese and the highland peasants of Jamaica as rare examples.

Khare (1986) comments that in India hospitality is based on values of duty, gifting, sacrifice and compassion. Obligatory hospitality appears between kin and jati members, social hospitality among friends, and alms-giving hospitality among those dispossessed, deprived and handicapped. The first is institutionalized; the second is casual and spontaneous, and the third is optional.

Food behaviour is thus a guide to both social relationships and to social structure. A rich tapestry of social meaning is woven around every food event in complex strands; assimilation of these meanings begins in childhood and so become an implicit part of adult behaviour and routine, understood and carried out without conscious thought or effort. Because food events may have more than one meaning depending on the actors and the circumstances of the play, some overlap will be apparent in the categories created below for purposes of discussion.

PRESTIGE AND STATUS

The table is the centre around which all reputations are formed.
De La Reynière (1968)

Historically, food has always been linked to social prestige and status. Some foods confer high status on the eaters, others assume high status because of the groups who habitually eat them. The discrepancy between the nobility and peasantry of Medieval England was exemplified by the contrast in their food intakes. While the poor sustained themselves with bread, cheese and other simple fare, nobles and landowners might sit down to suppers consisting of 20 or 30 different dishes, many of them containing meat of one kind or another. These grand feasts had a sociopo-litical purpose in that they symbolized the power which nobles held over the common people and also over food supplies. Meat was greatly desired by the general populace and in order to curb the common appetite and to maintain social distinctions several attempts were made to introduce sumptuary laws limiting the quality and quantity of foods which could be served. 'Meatless days' were proclaimed by law, but such legislation was largely unenforceable and other measures had to be adopted to preserve status differences. For example, the hunting of veni-son was forbidden to all but the nobility. In 19th century France, social position and food consumption were intimately connected. A gentleman was judged not by his wealth but by his knowledge and appreciation of the arts of the table.

In the modern world food continues to be a major way in which to assert social status. Prestige may be attached to foods themselves or to the circumstances and manner in which they are served. Pilau is eaten in India and Bangladesh by families of all socioeconomic status levels, but there are variations in type of fat used in the preparation. Wealthy fami-lies use ghee, middle-class families use shortening and poor families with access to coconut trees use coconut milk. Nice social distinctions can be subtly underlined through food behaviour or can be overtly stated by, for example, social rules which dictate who can eat with whom. High-caste Hindu Brahmins do not eat with untouchables; high-status medical consultants do not share the same dining room with low-status interns, or with nurses or dietitians. In many parts of the developing world it is traditional for the person with the highest prestige to eat first.

Some of the strictest rules governing who may eat with whom are enshrined in the Hindu caste system. These rules are linked with concepts of purity and pollution. What foods may be eaten by each caste and food exchanges between castes are also subject to control. Such prac-tices were largely derived from tribal customs which set peoples apart by the foods they accepted or rejected as food; inevitably, some food prac-tices came to be regarded as superior, as did the people who practised them. Eating habits thus became a mark of social rank which persists today, intrinsically bound to the economic and social systems of village India. Appadurai (1981) devized the concept of gastropolitics to analyse food behaviour as an expression of hierarchical relations among castes and symmetrical relations within subcastes. However, it should be noted that religious sects, which draw from all social backgrounds, may cut across regional and social caste ties.

Status and food behaviour

Impressing others through the vehicle of food events is a widespread method of asserting status. Eckstein (1980) says that status is conferred by freedom to choose rare and costly items to impress others; by freedom to select expensive restaurants for personal gratification; and by freedom to prepare difficult and time-consuming dishes. In Western society, freedom of choice is greatly prized, and to be denied a choice is nearly always viewed in a negative fashion. If one has a large array of choices then one has high status. The ability to choose freely is linked closely to economic factors; financial position has always been a measure of status and this is reflected in the goods and services which are purchased. Thus new cars, expensive paintings and exotic holidays have traditionally been symbols of wealth and status; they function by emphasizing the differences between those who have and those who have not. Lack of freedom to choose decreases self-esteem. Whenever food choice is restricted, most people will feel cheated and ill-at-ease. In institutions such as hospitals and schools food complaints are common and are at least partly attributable to the lack of freedom to choose; with therapeutic diets which severely limit food choice and yet are not life-threatening, there is a high rate of non-compliance – perhaps for very similar reasons. People living in impoverished circumstances, on social assistance or welfare, sometimes seem to make irrational choices by buying expensive luxury items, and are frequently criticized for extravagant behaviour. However, such behaviours provide an escape mechanism from the day-to-day reality of poverty, and have the effect of increasing self-esteem by creating the illusion of freedom of choice.

Status is also earned by the nature of the foods served. High status is attached to exotic foods, complex dishes and, usually, to expensive items – in which case the fact that the foods come largely from cans (caviar) or are prepared by someone else (servants) hardly matters; indeed, prestige may be enhanced by this distancing from actual food preparation. (As opposed to the low status of convenience or fast foods.) On the other hand, status may derive from the time and talent brought to bear on creating elaborate dishes. Perhaps here we can distinguish the 'good cook' from the 'good host', both of whom attract social kudos and thus acquire high status. As well as reflecting on the host's own status, the foods served at dinner parties can also be a comment on the status accorded to the guests. Thus for high-status guests more trouble is taken to prepare elaborate fare. The very question of who invites whom to dinner may be fraught with status implications. When the boss invites subordinates to dinner the social messages are quite different than when the subordinate invites the boss. At one time, before the era of raised consciousness toward sexism, it was almost impossible to open a popular magazine without seeing either an article or a cartoon which depicted a nervous and harassed wife caught in indecision over what to serve to her husband's boss in order to create just the right impression.

Food and fashion

Foods may assume a high status within a society simply because they are consumed by high-status groups. Historical examples of this are provided by the stories of white bread and white sugar. When white sugar first became available in Elizabethan England it was an expensive commodity which could only be afforded by the rich. It thus became a symbol of affluence and status to which others, lower in the social hierarchy, aspired in an attempt to elevate their own social standing. Once white sugar became widely used throughout all strata of society it lost its status value; brown sugar has now assumed the mantle of prestige. A similar pattern may be seen with white bread. As milling procedures became perfected white flour replaced the coarse dark flours which continued to characterize peasant status; everyone wanted white flour, despite its inferior nutritional value and taste. Cussler and DeGive (1952) comment that; 'changing the appearance of food usually involves complex techniques proportionate to the degree of civilization, so that highly milled and refined foods hold an approved position'. Even though it often looks like plaster-board and tastes like sponge, sliced, pre-packaged white bread has become widely desired. With this symbol of status undermined social leaders are now heading the movement back to wholemeal flours and breads. As a final historical example, consider dairy produce, which was known in Medieval and Tudor England as 'white meat' and which was eaten by people of all social classes but which, with the increasing prosperity of the 16th century, came to be regarded as inferior food fit only for the use of the common people (Drummond and Wilbraham, 1957). Ultimately it regained its general popularity, and came back into favour; throughout these vicissitudes of fashion the nutritional value of dairy produce remained exactly the same.

A modern example of feeding fashions, motivated at least partly by status considerations, is that of breastfeeding versus bottle feeding. When artificial milk formulae first became widely available commercially in the 1930s and 1940s they were eagerly promoted as an alternative to the near universal practice of breastfeeding, which as a natural function became degraded and 'low-class'. By the 1970s the social elite were spearheading the return to breastfeeding, claiming untold virtues for a practice which they once affected to despise. Bottle feeding persists among younger, less educated women from lower socioeconomic groups, who will no doubt in time also rediscover their biological capabilities. Meanwhile, in many parts of the developing world, an earlier phase of the cycle is still in evidence. Bottle feeding is perceived as being 'Northern' and 'modern' and therefore greatly to be desired. An extensive literature attests to the unsuitability of bottle feeding in conditions prevalent in rural areas of Africa, Asia and Latin America; yet families will expend large proportions of their total income to buy artificial formula milk. The often tragic consequences of this status seeking are seen in the awful toll of malnutrition and infant mortality.

Preferences may develop for high-status foods without regard to actual taste or nutritional value. De Garine (1976) examines food prestige among the Moussey, Massa and Toupouri tribes of Central Africa. He comments that only humans deliberately eschew the use of nutritionally valuable foods because they are considered to be of low status, and eat organoleptically mediocre or nutritionally poor foods in order to display economic prosperity. De Garine's fascinating account supports the view that the more societies are able to free themselves from subsistence and have at their disposal surpluses, the more food is used in a prestigious way. In our affluent societies we fret over what foods are 'in' and 'out'. The importance of prestige food lies in how much social recognition it confers, and the wrong choice could spell social disaster!

Status and food ownership

The above examples show how food consumption acts as a mark of status or as a symbol of the desire to rise in status. In some parts of the world food ownership has similar functions. In large parts of East, South and South-West Africa, cattle have an over-riding social and economic importance reflected in the fact that ownership of cattle is necessary if a man is to fully participate in social life. Without cattle he may be barred from certain rites of passage and be condemned to low social status. For example, among the Masai, bridewealth of ten cows must be paid to the father-in-law in order to obtain a wife. Cattle are kept as a symbol of wealth and status – a sort of bank account. They are also used to buy other goods and to pay fines. Although there is no actual prejudice against eating beef, the animals are not commonly killed for food. Simoons (1961) describes the cattle-keeping complex extant in sub-Saharan Africa. The Fulani of Nigeria regard cattle as symbols of wealth. Ownership of many cattle adds to a man's prestige so consequently cattle are rarely slaughtered except on special festive occasions. Elsewhere too, cattle have represented wealth; the word pecuniary is derived from a Latin root meaning riches in cattle. For the ancient Irish, Germans, Homeric Greeks and earliest Latins, cattle were the most important measure of wealth. The modern-day Western rancher who keeps large herds of steers is just as clearly demonstrating his wealth and status.

FOOD, FRIENDSHIP AND COMMUNICATION

Food is a universal medium for expressing sociability and hospitality. The closeness of social relationships between people might almost be gauged by the types of foods and meals they share together. A new neighbour may be invited for tea and biscuits; casual acquaintances attend a cheese and wine soiree; business associates are offered a buffet; close friends are invited to sit down and share a full meal. Douglas (1972) comments that a cocktail party which offers food is a bridge between the intimacy of meals and the distance of drinks, while Charles Merril Smith (1972) views it as a device for paying off obligations to people you don't want to invite for dinner. Food and drink is a part of most social functions, and even of more formal meetings, be it only tea or coffee and biscuits. The act of eating together indicates some degree of compatibility or acceptance. Food is offered as a gesture of friendship; the more elaborate the fare, the greater the implied intimacy or degree of esteem. Offering to share food is to offer to share a bit of oneself; to refuse food when offered is easily seen as a rejection of friendship. To accept an invitation to a social function and then to refuse the food is viewed as being unacceptable behaviour. Table 4.1 shows the importance of food, friendship and communication as enshrined in proverbs and sayings.

Table 4.1 Food and friendship in conventional wisdom

There is no joy in eating alone	The Buddha, 543 BC
War iyo la cuno, baa lagu nool yahay. Communication and food are the things that one lives by.	Somali proverb
An onion offered by a true friend is like a whole lamb.	Egyptian proverb
A crazy guest eats and leaves right away	Arabic proverb
He who shares my bread and salt is not my enemy	Bedouin proverb
Bana ba monna ba arolelana hloho ea tsie Children of a man share the head of a grasshopper (Relatives will share their food, no matter how little it is)	Sesotho proverb
Olugenda enjala teludda. A visitor who leaves with an empty stomach because you did not offer food will not easily return.	Ugandan proverb
Food for one person is enough for two, that for two is enough for four, that for four is enough for eight.	Islamic saying
Give the guest food to eat even though yourself are starving	Arab saying

It is common in European homes to always have a food item, usually something rich and sweet, to offer to casual callers. To not provide food is to fail socially and thus lose status. Similarly, Somalis consider it is poor manners not to offer visitors something to drink and householders prepare thermoses of hot spicy tea for the family and visitors throughout the day. Among the Kikuyu tribe of Kenya there is a basic assumption that every time you visit a home the host will feed you. Most visits are unannounced. It is impolite not to feed a visitor, and it is impolite for a guest to decline food that is offered. When people are travelling they may stop at any garden and eat without question. Only if they take food away is it considered stealing. Whenever special guests arrive in a Zairian home, it is important for the hosts to kill something or serve 'meat with blood'. Traditionally when they kill a chicken, they serve the entire chicken to the visitor who may then ask for any leftovers to take home or leave them for the host family to eat (Schlabach, 1991). For Haitians it is never polite to eat in the presence of others without offering some of your food. An unexpected guest who arrives when someone is eating may ask for some of the food without being considered rude. Haitians believe strongly that 'manje kwit pa gen met' – cooked food has no owner. Exceptionally, the Bemba people of Africa show their respect for a person not by inviting them to a meal, but instead sending food to be eaten in private. Among the Wamirans of Papua New Guinea, social etiquette centres on rules about food sharing. Any food that appears in public must be shared with as many people as see it. Food may be concealed, and the owner remain hungry, in order to avoid having to share. The most impolite behaviour is to intrude on someone who is getting, cooking or eating food as they must then immediately give some of it up (Kahn, 1986).

Peer acceptance

The social need to belong is an important motivator of human action. Food readily becomes an expression of the search for belongingness.

> As a lad he had grown up in a poor family of Italian origin. He was raised on blood sausage, pizza, spaghetti and red wine. After completing high school, he went to Minnesota and began working in logging camps where – anxious to be accepted – he soon learnt to prefer beef, beans, and beer, and he shunned all Italian food. Later, he went to a Detroit industrial plant and eventually became a promising young executive... In his executive role he found himself cultivating the favourite foods and beverages of other young executives; steak, whisky and sea-food. Ultimately he gained acceptance in the city's upper classes. Now he began winning admiration from people in his elite social set by going back to his knowledge of Italian food and serving them, with the aid of a manservant, authentic Italian treats such as blood-sausage, pizza, spaghetti and red wine.
>
> *Packard (1959)*

This quotation from Packard nicely illustrates the changing patterns of food uses and preferences in the attempt to fit in as social circumstances alter. The wish to eat what everyone else eats may result in very specific patterns, which sometimes raise issues of nutritional concern. A paramount example is that of teenagers and so-called 'junk foods'. For many teenagers and adolescents it is very important that while they dress and behave in ways which stress their non-identity with the adult world they do at the same time conform carefully to the expectations of their peer groups. This is equally true of food behaviour; if everyone else is drinking cola and eating burgers then it is a strong-minded teenager who chooses milk and salad. Food is often associated with meeting places; the coffee bar, the pub, the fish shop, the fast-food outlet. In each of these circumstances the appropriate food or drink is consumed. Schuchat (1973) aptly comments that eating is a social experience whereas nutrition is a health phenomenon. 'Junk food' is eaten in the context of a social experience which includes music, noise and company. In the structured home meal, where these elements are missing the teenager feels that the social experience has been denied.

Food choice in specific instances is governed by social niceties which may limit individual freedom to choose (though it is doubtful whether we often think of it in terms of peer pressure). For example, in a restaurant setting, once one person has chosen a soup and salad combination it is highly unlikely that others in the party will choose full three-course meals (Eckstein, 1980). It is unacceptable or, at least, embarrassing to be still eating long after everyone else has finished. In a recent BBC television drama a group of high-profile politicians have gathered to dine with the King of England and can hardly conceal their relish and anticipation as the hostess describes the Beef Wellington on the menu. Alas, when the King asks for just soup the other disappointed diners feel obliged to settle for the same.

Food as reward and punishment

The role of socialization in the acquisition of food habits has been discussed earlier; at that time we saw that attitudes to food could also be passed on in the socializing process. One of the specific ways in which children learn what is approved of and acceptable as food is through a system of reward and punishment. Rewards and punishments may be explicit or implicit and are often accompanied with other reinforcing messages. The child who has been good is rewarded with a chocolate bar; the ill-behaved child is sent to his or her room and deprived of supper. Concepts of good and bad which are quickly attached to foods through early social experiences with them may give rise to feeding problems which can and often do persist into adulthood. Margaret Mead has summed up these feelings and it is worth quoting her at some length. In contemporary America, she says:

> Resistances and acceptances of food are thought of in terms of morality. People feel that they ought to eat correctly, or, more

concretely 'It's wrong to eat too much sweet stuff'. Foods that are good for you are not good to eat, and foods that are good to eat are not good for you. So ingrained is this attitude that it may come as a surprise to learn that in many cultures there is no such contrast, that the foods which are thought to make people strong and well are also exclusively the foods which they like to eat, which they boast of eating, and without which they would be most unhappy.

Mead (1980)

Having made the point that it is indeed possible to choose 'wrong' foods, Mead continues:

Each generation of children is taught that bad food habits are a possibility against which they must continually be on guard. That is, traditionally, we have tried to make the correct consumption of foods an act of repetitive personal choice, instead of a semi-automatic behaviour. In many homes the 'right' food and the 'wrong' food are both placed on the table; the child is rewarded for eating the 'right' food and so taught that the right food is undesirable because, from the child's point of view, rewards are never given for doing things which in themselves are pleasurable or enjoyable. At the same time, children are punished by having the 'wrong' food taken away from them. Here again, the lesson is taught to the child that that which is delicious is an indulgence for which one is punished or with which one is rewarded. A dichotomy is set up in the child's mind between those foods which are approved and regarded by adults as undelicious and those foods which are disapproved but recognised as delightful. A permanent conflict situation is established which will remain with that child throughout life; each nutritionally desirable choice is made with a sigh, or rejected with a sense of guilt; each choice made in terms of sheer pleasure is either accepted with guilt or rejected with a sense of puritanical self-righteousness. Every meal, every food contact becomes an experience in which one must decide between doing right and enjoying oneself.

Probably, most parents have experienced the table-as-battleground syndrome at one time or another. It might be well to remind them that: (i) there is no special merit in consuming a particular vegetable or harm in omitting one which is disliked; (ii) children do have genuine dislikes; and (iii) that making the availability of one food contingent on the consumption of another is simply asking for trouble. Foods should be served in a positive family environment, and removed, if not eaten, with the least fuss possible. There is little sense in chastising a child for leaving on the plate those very same foods refused by Dad. Nutritionally acceptable desserts, incorporating fresh fruit and minimal sugar for example, can help avoid any necessity for the 'no pudding if you don't eat your dinner' gambit. As Mead indicates above, by insisting that a child remain at the table until the plate is clean, parents help to inculcate unhealthy attitudes and negative feelings about eating and meal times. Other studies have demonstrated that the use of foods in positive contexts as rewards or treats reinforces liking for them, whereas preferences are diminished for foods which have to be eaten in order to obtain a reward. Before parents protest too much about a conflict of theory and practice, it should be made very clear that eating and manners are quite separate affairs and that acceptable table behaviour, which is often what is desired of children, is not predicated on actual food consumption. Many food wars, I think, are due to confusion of the two.

FOOD GIFTS AND SHARING

'No matter how much food you have or how many guests you have, food will go around. When you share it, it goes around. It always does'. In Schlabach's world community cookbook stories like this one from Lesotho illustrate a recurring theme of how people with little food share it generously. In Haiti neighbours share food, sending it in covered dishes carried by children. At young ages, children imitate the customs of their parents, tearing off tiny portions of their 2-cent pieces of cassava bread to share with friends. Observation of food-sharing behaviour among American children at a summer camp revealed that items shared tended to be 'extras' rather than basic foods, and that they were used to establish friendships and cliques (Dyson-Hudson and van Dusen, 1972).

Food sharing has been studied as a psychological phenomenon too. Where children are reared in an environment of food abundance and their food needs are readily gratified, then a psychological predisposition to sharing is created (Cohen, 1961). The opposite is true in situations where food resources are scarce and where children are reared in an atmosphere of anxiety and deprivation.

Food is a universally acceptable gift by means of which the donor can express a variety of emotions such as concern, sympathy, or gratitude; food is frequently used to say 'you are loved...you are important'. Chocolate and other sweets are commonly used in this latter context. Mum gets a box of chocolates for her birthday; a sweetheart is presented with chocolates on Valentine's day; a hostess receives chocolates as a thank-you token for hospitality. Sometimes gifts have value in that they are home-made; a loaf of fresh bread, or a pot of country jam are personal tokens. At other times it is the cost or exotic value of foods which carries the social message; food hampers are popular gifts at Christmas, and usually contain delicacies and exotica rather than everyday foods. A gift is something given freely; a good or service for which no payment is required. It is true though that gift-giving is usually based on an unstated, but nevertheless expected, reciprocity. Three types of reciprocity may be identified each of which has different rules for exchanges.

Generalized reciprocity is characterized by exchanges which involve: (i) no immediate expectation of return; (ii) no attempt to assess the value of gifts; and (iii) no attempt to make gift-giving 'balance out'. That is records, mental or otherwise, are not kept. Generalized reciprocity occurs between family members and close friends in most societies. Balanced reciprocity, which occurs between people who are social equals and have some kind of personal relationship, does involve expectation of return (perhaps delayed), and takes account of the value of the gift. Thus in some commercial concerns smoked hams, bottles of whisky, or wine may be given to valued customers at Christmas time in the expectation that the gift will be reciprocated through continued business orders. Similarly, sales agents entertain clients to dinner, offering a meal in exchange for a contract. An invitation to supper is issued with the general expectation that the hospitality will be returned at a later date; if it is not, then social relations may be damaged or even terminated. A well-understood social code such as this is open to deliberate manipulation. For example; a middle-manager invites the director to supper where she has the chance to impress and flatter her boss by serving an elaborate meal. Under the rules of reciprocity, the manager later attends a supper at the director's house, thereby increasing her own status in the eyes of others. Negative reciprocity involves immediate exchange and strict accounting of value; the exchange is impersonal (Hardisty, 1977). Commercial transactions typify this kind of exchange.

Food exchanges can also be ways of expressing friendship while maintaining economic parity; exchanges diffuse the status meanings of a food event. Thus wine may be given in exchange for a meal, an arrangement which allows guests to contribute and to establish a feeling of mutual friendship, while relieving some of the economic burden placed on the hosts. Another view of this exchange process might see it as lessening obligations on the part of the meal's recipients. Having been wined and dined at the expense of another, a guest may feel to have been placed under an obligation to the hosts. Offerings of wine, for example, repay this obligation on the spot. The potluck dinner is another example of mutual exchange which allows sociability without status or obligation considerations intruding; each guest contributes to the overall meal and also shares in the gifts bought by others.

Sharing the harvest is a way of ensuring community food security for Peruvian Indian societies. If some families do not harvest sufficient to eat, the community organizes an ancient feast called kausay huñuy which means 'collecting food to promote life'. The feast takes place in the home of the needy family, one member of which is appointed as the aqakamoyog or host. She prepares chicha, a strong corn drink, and spreads out a huge shawl on the patio where the food will be collected. As neighbours come by, the aqakamoyog gives them a glass of chicha; after they leave their food gift she gives them two more glasses. Word spreads quickly that this family is serving good chicha, thus encouraging others to come and share. When the shawl is full, the family gathers round to bless the crop and give thanks. Kausay huñuy embodies the solidarity expressed in a common saying 'today this is for you: tomorrow it may be for me' (Rodriguez, 1986). Some rural food banks in Canada adopt a similar philosophy. When times are good you contribute food to the food bank; when times are bad, you take what you need.

Charitable food sharing and rationing

Although food sharing is a major feature of hospitality it also occurs through charitable sentiments and mechanisms. Charitable food giving is usually an optional, voluntary activity as compared with hospitality which is formally or informally governed by social expectations. Receiving food charity may be interpreted by both donors and recipients as a form of alms-giving or as begging and as such may be damaging to self-esteem, honour and prestige. 'People do not want to give away food in charity when they face scarcity themselves, and most people do not like to receive food as "alms", though in need. Some give food but only with "strings"; and while some receive it with indifference, others take it as a matter of right. Some give food to assert their social status and privileges while others do so to express equality and nearness. Some dispute the giver's status and privilege even as they accept his food.' (Firth, 1967).

In India there is a moral duty to feed others generously, which helps restrain any sense of superiority on the part of donors or alienation of recipients (Khare, 1986). Still, people may avoid charity, even when facing scarcity, because of the risk to their social honour. In Canada, food banks and soup kitchens act as channels of charitable food distribution and are viewed ambivalently by donors and recipients alike. Food bank users often express feelings of low self-esteem or loss of dignity.

Just as food hospitality blurs into charity, so charity blurs into rationing. State-administered feeding programmes and rationing schemes (such as school meals and food stamps) recognize human entitlements to food, whereas charity depends on moral duty. During times of deprivation and hardship, such as caused by war, government-administered rationing is a policy tool used to ensure that everyone has a sufficient share of scarce foodstuffs.

Sharing, competition and scarce resources

Food exchanges based on some form of reciprocity principle are common in situations where environmental resources are limited and where it would be disastrous to encourage intensive productive effort. This is the case with forager cultures, where a low and irregular work effort is best suited to ecological conditions. Generalized reciprocity helps to maintain this low-level activity and to prevent excessive exploitation of the environment in attempts to gain social status. It ensures that no-one boasts about their generosity in gift-giving, which would create a social atmosphere conducive to status competition and which in turn would stimulate extra work and intensive resource exploitation. In instances where reciprocity has not been adopted, the use of food as a means of establishing social status has in several societies given rise to the practice of competitive food giving. Among the Massim of New Guinea food giving is a form of social control. Wrongdoers are given more food than they are able to return – which draws attention to the transgression and restores honour to the victim (Young, 1971). Perhaps though, the ultimate example of 'fighting with food' is to be found in the North American Indian ceremony known as potlatch.

Potlatch

Potlatch was the name given to great feasts of the North-West Coast Indians in which the giving away of material wealth was a central occurrence. The name potlatch was derived from the Nootka verb Pa-chitle – to give, and the noun Pa-chuck – article to be given, and thus described the specific type of festival in which public gift-giving occurred. The potlatch has been regarded by some as being merely an extravagant and wasteful display of wealth in which prestige is gained at the cost of material impoverishment (Hou, 1973). In contrast to this view, Bozak (1973) says that potlatch feasts symbolized religious, ethical and legal concepts and were an important functional part of Indian society. Also, by accepting food and gifts at these feasts, guests acknowledged the host's status.

Potlatches commonly celebrated major life-events such as birth, puberty, marriage and death; elaborate festivals signified the death of a great chief. Other potlatches were termed 'face-saving'; by giving a feast, an individual who had suffered embarrassment or misfortune or who had offended against social law, could redeem himself and maintain his position in society (Rohner and Rohner, 1970). Then there were penalty potlatches, imposed on those who breached ceremonial taboos; for example, laughing, stumbling or coughing at winter dances. Whatever the motivation for the potlatch, it was always a public rather than private affair. The host, with the support of his family, clan or tribe invited members of other tribes to witness his actions and claims. The guests legitimized the use of any songs, dances or other privileges claimed by the host. Dancing, feasting, speech-making and gift-giving occupied the time. During the potlatch, gifts were distributed according to the rank of the guests. Food, money, property – all could be and were given.

Originally, gifts were handmade or home produced, but these were eventually superseded by manufactured wares obtained through trading with White men. Guests were shamed by the large amounts of wealth given to them and immediately started to plan their own potlatches in which the wealth could be returned, with interest. Though it might take many years to accumulate sufficient wealth to be able to give a potlatch, this wealth was sometimes conspicuously destroyed simply to add to the grandeur of the occasion; canoes were burnt, and blankets and precious sheets of copper destroyed, all in the pursuit of gaining status.

The collection, storage and preparation of food prior to the festival was of great importance; many delicacies would be painstakingly gathered and prepared. In addition to the food needed for gifts, meals had to be served every day of the ceremony which commonly lasted for one full phase of the moon. Food was served generously and excess was taken home by visitors to eat later or to share with those who did not attend the feast. It was important to ensure that no-one was left out, and it would have been a source of great shame if guests had been able to eat everything provided. The potlatch was a means of sharing: 'your good fortune, wealth, affluence with fellow men...be it your worldly belongings, your food or your goodwill...' (Clutesi, 1969).

The government of the White settlers held a different view. They could not understand the ceremonial functions of potlatching and saw only the poverty and destitution which descended on those who had given away all their possessions. In fact, potlatches were usually reciprocated by the guests, and they acted as a means of redistribution of wealth among the tribes – similar to that seen in some African societies. Different tribes lived in different environments of river, coast and woods; in any given year the food harvest in one area might be prolific while in another region food could be scarce. By holding a potlatch a rich tribe could share its bounty with others not so well off, at the same time accumulating much prestige and status (Suttles, 1960). The Kwakiutl West Coast Indians, for example, were organized into local kinship groups, known as numaym, which owned fishing locations, hunting territories, houses and goods. They were led by a chief who was custodian of the resources and who performed rituals; each numaym was self-sufficient and not tied to other groups. When the microenvironment changed so that resource availability declined, for example when ocean currents moved salmon runs to other coastal areas, self-sufficiency was endangered and warfare sometimes resulted. More often though, surplus food from other numaym could be obtained in exchange for material wealth such as blankets and canoes. Competitive feasting, by stimulating resource production, was a way of ensuring that one group would have a food surplus so that this exchange could take place. If a famine was prolonged and a numaym exhausted its material wealth, it could still obtain food in exchange for social status (Hardisty, 1977).

Farb and Armelagos (1980) see the potlatch as an adaptive behaviour which provided the setting and reason for exchange of resources, as well as encouraging high food productivity in readiness for the next feast. Rivalry and prestige were not the moving principles, but rather excuses for keeping the potlatch going. However, in 1884, a law was enacted which forbade direct or indirect involvement with potlatching on pain of imprisonment (LaViolette, 1973). It proved impossible to consistently enforce this law; in time, the positive values of the potlatch came to be more appreciated and it was recognized as being an important event for expressing respect and honour, for entertainment and for sharing resources. In 1951 the potlatch law was abolished but by this time there had been considerable changes in Indian culture and the potlatch never regained its former prominence and glory.

Because the Indian potlatch is carried out within the context of an unfamiliar culture and is strikingly overt in its competitive aims it may be classified as an irrational and alien practice. However, de Garine (1970) comments that most meals on social occasions are held in a spirit of competition, with each group attempting to outdo the others, though in post-industrial societies quality is usually more important than quantity. European wedding feasts are cited as an example. Conspicuous consumption and prestige economies are still very important in many developing countries, as illustrated in examples already cited in earlier sections of this chapter. Harris (1974) adds that among peoples who do not have a defined ruling class, competitive feasting is a near universal mechanism for assuring production and distribution of wealth within the society.

FEASTS AND FESTIVALS

The word feast denotes a special occasion, commonly public, on which food is consumed of a different quality and quantity to that of everyday meals. In many places the feast is a community event with no exclusive guest list; everyone is welcome.

In general, the foods used for feasting are: (i) scarce; (ii) high quality; (iii) often expensive; and (iv) difficult and time-consuming to prepare. That is, they have high status. They are definitely different from the everyday fare. Meat is often a preferred component in the diet but most people in the world can only afford it on special occasions. In South African Xhosa society, meat is reserved for occasions, such as birthdays, marriages, deaths and farewells, that draw enough people together to consume an entire animal. The exclusive tie between eating meat and festive occasions is so strong that people refer to these occasions as times when they 'eat meat'. In Lesotho a mokete or feast must have meat, so people plan and host feasts at times when that is possible. If there is an unexpected funeral, for example, a meatless funeral meal is served, but another feast is hosted later when the hosts are able to kill and share an animal (Schlabach, 1991).

Festivals are complex and colourful events, being forms of ritual found in practically every society in one guise or another. They are public events which may be of a religious or secular nature, and which usually include feasting as part of more general celebrations. Often they occur at vital points in the human and cosmic lifecycle and themselves incorporate a cycle of events which represent or reflect the society's philosophy of history (Crim, Bullard and Shinn, 1981). Thus themes of birth and death, decay and renewal, sowing and reaping, summer and winter, are common. Four major types of festival can be distinguished. Ecofests celebrate astronomical or seasonal events and are frequently associated with pre-literate or pagan rituals which were designed to ensure control of the food supply. Theofests celebrate religious events and are often wedded to ecofest predecessors; for example, Christmas celebrates the birth of Christ and also the winter solstice. Many festivals had an agrarian origin, but as they became associated with particular events or deities they ceased to be seasonal as such. As well, new festivals were instituted which had none of the agrarian rationale of earlier celebrations; instead, they celebrated national, local and political occasions. These may be labelled, as a third group, secular festivals. A fourth category of festival embraces personal rituals; into this grouping can be placed birthdays and anniversaries, together with rites of passage such as weddings and funerals. Brief accounts of some different types of festivals are given below, together with a list of festivals around the world (Table 4.2).

Celebrated in many parts of the world, May Day is a good example of an ecofest. It originally represented pagan attempts to force spring to return to the world, and was focused on themes of freshness and renewal. Cosman (1981) describes the medieval uses of green foods at this celebration; green parsley bread slices, green salads, green fruit and green apple cider: green peppermint rice and minted green whipped cream – all representative of the victory of spring after the barren winter months. Halloween marks the end of the ancient Celtic year, the division between the end of summer and the beginning of winter. It also precedes the church holiday of All Saint's Day and the following All Soul's Day. On this latter day, prayers were offered up for the souls waiting in Purgatory, a practice introduced by Odilo, Abbot of Cluny in 998 AD, but abolished in England during the Reformation, though it survived among continental Protestants. It is essentially an adaptation of an almost world-wide custom of setting aside part of the year for the dead. Historically, children would beg for soul cakes (shortbread biscuits with currants, cinnamon and nutmeg) for the wandering spirits. If no cakes were offered then the souls would play pranks. This custom is of course continued in the trick or treat visits of North American children to neighbours' houses on Hallowe'en. The householder gives sweets, candies or other food treats to

Table 4.2 Festivals around the world

Date		Name	Country	Type
January	6	Epiphany	Various	T
	25	Robbie Burns Night	Scotland	N
February	14	St. Valentine's Day	Various	TP
March		Easter	Various	ET
	19	Feast of St. Joseph	Italy	T
	21	New Year	Persia	E
April	1	All Fool's Day	Various	T
May	1	May Day	Various	ET
	5	Children's Day	Japan	P
	14	Independence Day	Israel	N
June	24	Midsummer Day	Various	E
	24	St. John's Day	Brazil	ET
July	25	Feast of St. James	Spain	N
August	15	Assumption of Mary	Various	T
September	29	Michaelmas	Various	T
October		Octoberfest	Germany	N
	14	Thanksgiving	Canada	ET
	31	Hallowe'en	N. America	E
November	1	All Saints' Day	Various	T
	2	All Souls' Day	Various	ET
	5	Guy Fawkes' Night	Britain	N
	20	Anniversary of the Revolution	Mexico	N
December	5	Sinterklaas	Holland	P
	13	St. Lucia Day	Sweden	T
	25	Christmas	Various	ET
	31	Hogmanay	Scotland	N

E, Ecofest; T, Theofest; ET, eco + theofest; N, National; P, Personal
N.B. This classification is not rigid; many festivals have multiple origins

placate these modern day spirits or else risks becoming the victim of (usually) harmless pranks. In Italy, All Soul's Day is celebrated with feasting in remembrance of loved ones.

Christmas is celebrated in varying ways and on varying days in many places throughout the world. Although it is predominantly a religious festival it is blended with older pagan and agrarian customs. (In a similar way, many churches were built on the sites of earlier pagan worshippers.) Indeed, the extent to which religions can adopt and adapt existing practices may account largely for their survival and spread. For example, when Sweden became a Christian country in 1537 the Church immediately assimilated certain pagan traditions. Lussi, the Queen of Light, was linked to the Italian St. Lucia and celebration of St Lucia's Day now marks the beginning of Christmas festivities in Sweden. The pagan custom of feeding birds and animals to ensure fertility in the coming year is continued in Baltic and Slavic countries where, on Christmas Eve, bread and barley is fed to farm animals before the family eats its own evening meal. On Christmas morning in Jos, Nigeria, people send bowls of prepared chicken stew and rice to each other. In the afternoon, women go singing and dancing from house to house where they share grain drinks and meat, rice and sweets prepared for the occasion. In New Zealand a traditional Christmas dinner is served in the winter month of June, as December 25th is more likely to be spent sun-tanning on the beach and is hardly suited to turkey and all the trimmings.

Christmas is an example of a festival which has spread around the world even though it has not always retained its original meaning. The Bushmen of Africa hold a special feast and dance for Christmas; their knowledge of Christmas originated from the London Missionary Society's work in Africa and, according to Lee (1969) they view it as being a celebration to 'praise the birth of white man's god-chief'. At this time a great ox is slaughtered by the Tswana headman and distributed among the bushmen. Lee describes the difficulties he encountered when, having lived with the Bushmen for some time, he tried to donate the festive ox. In other parts of the world, the religious meaning of Christmas is being deliberately eroded. In pre-breakup Russia, Christmas was symbolized by the confrontation between Grandfather Frost and the villainous Baba Yaga; nationalist plays, songs and dances were performed in which Grandfather Frost, aided by the Young Pioneers, defeated his evil adversary (Barer-Stein, 1979).

Easter is widely celebrated as a religious festival often spreading over several weeks, though Easter Sunday and the week preceding have become the focus of modern Easter celebrations. It was named for the pagan Goddess Eostre, the Goddess of dawn and Spring, and occurred at the time of the Spring Equinox in March. The cycle of celebration heralded the triumph of light over dark; of summer over winter. Echoes of the pagan ecofest are seen in the traditional Hot Cross Buns served at Easter. The cross represents the four seasons, while the round bun itself is the sun.

Religious festivals abound in the Hindu calendar. In Southern India certain foods are offered to specific deities and are specific to particular festivals. Pure deities may only accept vegetarian food. In the 18 major Hindu festivals, special foods are featured; rice and bananas symbolize fertility; ghee (clarified butter) symbolizes purity, and coconut and mango symbolize sacredness and auspiciousness (Katona-Apte, 1976). Other examples of religious festivals are given in Chapter 6.

National holidays mark events in the history of a peoples or in the lives of notable figures. The well-known German Oktoberfest originated as a holiday to celebrate the wedding of Crown Prince Ludwig in 1810. Scots the world over pay homage to the poet Robbie Burns on the anniversary of his birth, January 25th, with a feast featuring the ethnic delicacy known as haggis. Many countries include feasting in their Independence Day celebrations.

Folklorama is the name of an annual festival held each year in Winnipeg, Manitoba, to celebrate the rich diversity of cultures which make up that city. For 2 weeks in the summer over 40 ethnic groups provide food, entertainment and cultural displays in a series of pavilions throughout the city. Food is one of the main attractions and visitors can buy snacks, single dishes or whole meals. In some cases dishes are altered to appeal to mainstream North American tastes, but mostly they are traditional recipes which offer a genuine ethnic food experience (Table 4.3).

Table 4.3 Food at Folklorama

Pavilion	Foods offered
Belgian	Belgian waffles; vinken
Caribbean	Jerk pork; roties
Chilean	Curanto; torte mil hojas
Down-Under	Chilled kiwi and mango soup; damper
French–Canadian	Tortière; pea soup
German	Bratwurst; sauerkraut
Greek	Souvlaki; moussaka; baklava
Hungarian	Szekely goulash; langosh
India	Curry; rice pulao; gulab jaman
Israeli	Kugel; blintzes; gefillte fish
Japan	Sushi; temura; teriyaki chicken
Metis	Buffalo stew; bannock
Portuguese	Squid; octopus
Scandinavian	Inlagd sild; vinaterte
Scottish	Haggis; mealy puddings
Ukrainian	Varenky; kovbasa
Vietnamese	Spring rolls; spicy chicken

Folklorama demonstrates the integral role of food in maintaining and promoting cultural identity. Although some of the 'national' dishes offered (e.g. Scottish haggis) may not exactly be accurate reflections of homeland eating habits they do illustrate the importance of the idea of a national heritage cuisine. Food at Folklorama acts as a vehicle for introducing people to other cultural traditions; it provides a necessary element in a social event, as strangers sit together to share. It is also a focus for

Social functions of food

Table 4.4 Wedding feast of Henry IV

First course
    Braun en peuerade   Slices of meat cooked in spiced sweet sauce
    Viaund Ryal   Puree of rice and mulberries sweetened with
                               honey, flavoured with wine and spices

    Test de senglere
    enarmez   Boar's head and tusks
    Graunde chare   Large piece of roasted meat
    Syngettys   Cygnets
    Capoun de haute grece   Capon à la foie gras geese
    Fesaunte   Pheasants
    Heroun   Heron
    Crustarde Lumbarde   Pie of cream, eggs, dates, prunes and sugar
    Storieoun graunt luces   Sturgeon and great pike
    Subtlety

Second course
    Venyson en furmenty   Venison served with a spiced grues of cream,
                               wheat and eggs
    Gely   Calves foot jelly with white wine and vinegar
    Porcelle farce enforce   Stuffed suckling pigs
    Pokokkys   Peacocks served in their plumage
    Cranys   Cranes
    Venyson roste   Roast venison
    Conyng   Rabbits over a year old
    Byttore   Bitterns
    Pulle endore   Glazed chicken
    Graunt tartez   Great pies of meat, game and poultry
    Braun fryez   Fritters of meat
    Leche Lumbard   Spiced date cakes
    Subtlety

Third course
    Blaundesorye   Almond and chicken mousse
    Quyneys in comfyte   Quinces preserved in syrup
    Egretes   A kind of heron
    Curlewys   Curlews
    Pertrych   Partridges
    Pyionys   Pigeons
    Quaylys   Quails
    Snytys   Snipe
    Rabettys   Young rabbits
    Smal Byrdys   Small birds
    Pome Dorreng   Rissoles of pork roasted on a spit, basted with
                               spices and herbs
    Braun blanke leche   Meat in white sauce
    Eyroun engele   Eggs in jelly
    Frytourys   Fritters
    Doucettys   Custard tarts
    Pety perneux   Small spiced tarts of eggs, cream and raisins
    Subtlety

*Based on information from Drummond, J.C and Wilbraham, A. (1957) *The Englishman's Food*, Revised edition, Jonathan cape, London

maintaining a sense of community within the larger community of Winnipeg, as people come together to plan, prepare and serve the food of their homeland.

Personal celebrations usually revolve around major life events. The Greek writer, Herodotus, says the custom of birthdays was well established among ancient Persians of rank. Modern birthday parties call forth special birthday foods, often in the form of sweet treats, jellies and cakes. In Japan, birthday celebrations include the serving of lobster; the hump of the lobster represents the bent back of old age and by partaking of it the celebrant is desired of living to an old age. In Korea, a child's first birthday is an occasion for special celebration. The infant is dressed in bright clothes and given rice cakes, fruit and cookies; he or she is placed in the midst of symbols which represent possible future careers and onlookers try to guess which one the child will grasp first.

Wedding feasts, although perhaps not always as elaborate as the royal meal described in Table 4.4, are prepared with particular care. Wedding cake is traditionally shared out among guests so that blessings and happiness can be shared. Sometimes, the top tier of the wedding cake is kept to be used at the christening of the first child. On the day before a Lebanese wedding, guests are served sweet pastries, nuts and candy-coated almonds as a symbol of a sweet and prosperous life. At a middle-class Sunni Muslim marriage feast the bride's father is expected to offer food and hospitality to a large group of relatives friends and neighbours, the number of guests being a matter of prestige and social obligation. The feast acts both to publicize the marriage and reinforce social bonds. Many Muslims are members of occupational brotherhoods called biradarīs; where this is the case there is an expectation that the entire local segment of the biridarī will be invited. Pennypinching would dishonour the family and imply denial of proper hospitality to the community, so that the cost of food is a major wedding expense. 'This seems to be an example of economic rationality being subjected to an economy of symbols' (Murphy, 1986). To reduce the burden of cost some biradarīs have banned members from giving wedding meals; instead guests get tea and light snacks. However, to qualify as a feast, meat dishes must be offered, and prestige is a function of the number of dishes and high status types of meat. Muslim hosts are faced with a dilemma in inviting Hindu friends to wedding feasts; the hosts know that many Hindus are meat-eaters who enjoy Muslim meat dishes, but they also know that normative patterns for some Hindu castes prohibit meat. Usually, separate arrangements are made for vegetarian guests, including the hiring of Hindu Brahmin cooks.

Feasts are commonly held to honour the dead. Homer describes in the Iliad how King Priam ends the funeral for his slain son, Hector, with a banquet – an early example of a wake. In many Western countries, it is traditional after a burial service to invite guests back to a funeral meal prepared by relatives and friends of the deceased. In Gitksan society, food was burned on cremation pyres; food was also put into the hands of a corpse, and in gravehouses to feed the deceased's afterlife self in the Beyond. It was believed that when a burning log hissed, the dead were signalling their presence and usually their need of food. Someone immediately responded by tossing a little bit of food into the fire. The contemporary term used for flowers given at funerals literally means 'to make a pack lunch for someone other than yourself to take on a journey' (People of 'Ksan, 1980).

These examples illustrate the variety and wide extent of festivals in marking the events held to be important in a society. In the next section, we examine a different type of ritual event – the sacrifice.

RITUALS AND SACRIFICE

When we speak of something having been ritualized we envisage a repetitive act carried out in a codified manner. Thus we can point to the morning ritual of shower, newspaper and breakfast; or to the cinematic ritual of popcorn, ice cream and soft drinks. More often, we think of rituals as connoting religious or supernatural activities. They permit the expression of sentiments which can not always be put into words and can thus act as a unifying social force. Many rituals, both pagan and religious, involve food in some way. Indeed, the need for particular foods for use in rituals may have contributed to their spread throughout different parts of the world. Thus Hindus needed tumeric, Christians needed wine and Jews needed citron; when these peoples migrated they took their ritual foods with them (Isaac, 1959). Rituals often involved some kind of offering. Food offerings, which in modern civilizations may be of a plant nature, were previously almost always animal in nature. For example, the Brahman sacrifices of rice cakes were actually substitutes for human beings. Abrahams' substitution of a ram for his son Isaac, indicates that Hebrews were aware of the custom of human sacrifice and of its substitution by animal. Animal sacrifice was a well-established mode of religious worship, though as life became more urbanized even this was discontinued by the Israelites, and instead they were able to purchase redemption with silver. Eventually it was declared that fasting and prayer would be sufficient; loss of bulk through fasting could be seen as being equivalent to sacrificial offerings in that it represented a 'giving up' of self, while 'He who prays is considered as pious as if he had built an altar and offered sacrifices upon it.' (Harris, 1923). This evolutionary pattern of sacrificial offering: human – animal/plant – money – prayer: is repeated in the history of many societies. Candles, incense and money offerings in modern churches echo primitive offerings of flesh and blood (Tannahill, 1976).

An offering is a species of gift and as such it must have certain characteristics. It should be personal, that is something owned rather than a gift of nature; it should have value for the giver and it should be given voluntarily. Sacrifice implies an asymmetrical status relationship. While a gift puts the recipient in an inferior social position, an offering emphasizes that it is the giver who is of inferior status (Firth, 1965). Sacrifices may be offered for a number of different reasons:

- As food for the Gods
- To propitiate an affronted deity
- To communicate with a deity by eating of sacrificial victim (omophagy)
- For maintenance or renewal of life
- For divination purposes
- To confirm a covenant
- To ward off evil
- In exchange for favours

The custom of offering something to a deity is ancient and widespread; it is an instinctive part of human nature. Food, as a gift of the Gods, is sacred, and most cultures have particular rituals or procedures to de-sanctify the first crop in order to make it suitable for ordinary humans. Offering food shows devotion to a supernatural force, and in all rural societies, offering of first fruits is practised (de Garine, 1970).

Sir Edward Tylor (1871) regarded sacrifice as being essentially a gift to the supernatural being to minimize its hostility. Homeric Greeks occasionally killed prisoners to placate an angry God, and Romans made sacrifices of Greeks and Christians. More often animal sacrifices were used, until with time such gifts developed into homage then abnegation as described above.

The anthropologist W. Robertson-Smith viewed sacrifice as a communion between members of a group, and between them and their God. Sacrifice acted as a buffer between the sacred deity and the profane human, thus avoiding any dangerous direct contact. Cannibalistic elements arose because by eating a portion of the sacrifice humans identified themselves with what was being offered to the Gods. Sometimes the sacrifice symbolized the deity itself so the eaters could in this way absorb the Divine. Frazer saw these rituals as a kind of magic in which the sacrifice was a way of rejuvenating a God. Kill the God to save him from decay and to aid his rebirth; kill a victim to feed and strengthen the God; kill the rivals of the God to facilitate his resurrection (Frazer, 1963). The Creation myth and Resurrection myth were dominant in primitive religions and these original dramas had to be re-enacted each year by the Gods with the help of man. To aid the return of the fertility deity to the soil the farmer contributed strength and power in the form of human sacrifice (Tannahill, 1976). Such sacrifices persist; the Aymaras of Bolivia ritually kill llamas and sprinkle their blood on newly planted potatoes (Heiser, 1990).

Animals have often been used for divination arts. The entrails of a sacrifice would be examined and from this great prophecies made. Andean Indians sacrificed llamas and examined their lungs and entrails for omens. Cattle and sheep were sacrificed at the Temple of Solomon as an act of repentance and in fulfilment of vows. A well-known biblical example of sacrifice designed to ward off ill is the Israelite sacrifice of the Paschal lamb, whose blood was smeared on doors so that the Israelites would be spared when the Egyptians were smitten by the death of their first-born.

Normally when sacrifices are made no material counter-gifts are expected. However, subsequent fertility of crops or personal health may be ascribed to such sacrifice. Bantu offer domesticated animals (not wild ones, for they are a free gift of nature and have lower status) in return for demands for the spirit's blessing. The Nuer of southern Sudan make offerings which then 'obligate' the Gods to return the favour. Many agri-culturalist peoples made blood sacrifices, including human sacrifices, to ensure a good crop. The modern Harvest Festival custom of placing an old grain among the new, parallels the blood and ashes added to corn in past times (Firth, 1965).

There is little waste in sacrifice. Priests, responsible for officiating at sacrifices, often lived off what was offered to the Gods. Frequency and quality of sacrifice are affected by economics in that there is a relation between what is offered and resource availability. If animals are scarce then excuses can be found for not having a sacrifice. In the case of the Nuer of Sudan, if prize cattle cannot be spared then older infirm cattle, sheep, goats or even cucumbers are substituted. When cattle sacrifices are made, then meat is shared in the village. Economic calculations have been ever present in human affairs, and when the offerer can substitute something less valuable for the sacrifice, he does so, using a variety of rationales for his action. Indeed, the value of the thing offered is attributed to it only conventionally by virtue of its being selected for offering. A more jaundiced view is offered by Marvin Harris who interprets the end of animal sacrifice as signifying the end of ecclesiastical redistributive feasting, and the move to Heavenly worship as being a means of slipping out of responsibilities to provide for people on earth. Thus the open-handed generosity of barbaric chiefs who held great feasts and fed their followers was eschewed by Christianity, Buddhism and Islam, whose leaders were transformed from great providers to great believers – and who served nothing to eat in their temples (Harris 1977).

Sacraments

Many cultures, particularly ancient ones, have had their sacred foods. Frazer points out that a sacred animal is often an embodiment of the God himself. Attis of Phrygia was, according to legend, killed by a wild boar. The pig was identified with Attis and was thereafter not eaten by his followers. However, ritual sacrifices could be made of the pig so that the believers could consume their God sacramentally. The sacramental killing and eating of an animal implies that the animal is sacred and is as a rule spared. The Greek writer Herodotus said that the ancient Egyptians looked upon the pig with loathing. No one would touch a pig, drink of its milk or have social intercourse with swineherds and their families. However, once a year, pigs were sacrificed to the Moon and Osiris, and the flesh was eaten. Frazer supposes that this was a sacramental meal and that the pig was a sacred animal (Frazer, 1963; paragraph 373). He supports this by alluding to the fact that in many belief systems it is not permitted to touch sacred objects in the normal course of everyday life.

There are parallels, noted by early anthropologists, between the Christian Eucharist and primitive sacrifices. At the Last Supper Jesus had said 'Take; this is my body' and 'This is my blood of the covenant' (Mark 14:22–24). In the original Eucharist, or Thanksgiving, the community gave thanks as they ate bread from the same loaf and drank wine from the same cup, thus commemorating the death of Jesus. St Paul, anxious for potential converts among Jews, Romans, Greeks and Pagans, presented the Last Supper as a sacrifice in which Jesus was the Paschal lamb who was offered up. Because of the calendrical proximity of the two events Paul was easily able to transfer the symbolism of Passover to the Crucifixion. St Paul seems to have been responsible for instituting the custom of re-enactment of the sacrifice by emphasizing the words 'do this in remembrance of me' as Jesus' instructions at the Last Supper. Only the gospel of Luke includes these words, and they were written at a time after Paul's correspondence with the Greeks in which he had urged the ritual re-enactment. Also, Luke was a close friend of Paul (Tannahill, 1976). Out of these adjustments was born the ritual of the Mass. From an early time some men, like St. John Chrystostom, Archbishop of Constantinople, believed in transubstantiation, while most continued to view the mass as a symbolic act. A conflict, or at least an inconsistency, arose which threatened to weaken the concept of Papal supremacy. The Medieval Church wanted to wield temporal as well as spiritual power and there was no room in it for dissent; all had to submit absolutely to the will of God. Hence Pope Innocent III determined to resolve the dispute. In 1215 CE Innocent held the assembly of the Fourth Lateran Council where the Catholic church decreed that when a priest pronounced 'This is my body' at Mass, then the bread and wine were truly changed to the body and blood of Christ. The Host was no longer a symbol but an

actuality, and to deny this was heresy. The Communion was thus transformed from being a symbolic act to an equivalent of the pagan rituals of
omophagy, or eating of the God. The Communion loaf was later replaced
by unleavened wafers when it was realized that, as a Jew, Jesus would
not have eaten leavened bread during Passover. Tannahill (1976) gives an
account of how the red bacíllus which sometimes grew on stale food was
misinterpreted as being bleeding of the Host. Because the Host was so
closely identified by Christians as the body of Christ ('Host' is derived
from Latin 'Hostia', meaning sacrificial victim), the conclusion was
reached that it was being tortured by Jews who had, after all, crucified
Jesus through their hate of him. This resulted in massive persecutions of
Jews in the 13th and 14th centuries.

SUMMARY

Truly, food usages are signposts to understanding different cultures.
Patterns of food preparation, distribution and consumption reflect the
dominant type of social relationships in a society. They are an expression
of status and social distance, of political power and of family bonds. Food
is extensively used in social intercourse as a means of expressing friendship and respect. The quality and quantity of food offered or shared
reflects a common understanding of the closeness of various types of
social relationships. Food is also used as a manipulative tool to purchase
favours or to bring about desired behaviours, and as a weapon with
which to humiliate rivals. It confers status through ownership or usage,
and is commonly a part of ritual proceedings. Food is an indispensable
element in festivals and celebrations where it may be again symbolic of
social relationships or where it may assume supernatural powers.

FURTHER READING

For a delightful account of Medieval celebrations the reader is referred to
Cosman (1981).
Thelma Barer-Stein (1979) gives extensive details of festivals and tradi-
tional foods among ethnic groups in Canada, in *You Eat What You Are*,
McClelland & Stewart, Toronto.
For detailed discussions of the Hindu caste system, see:
Hasan, K.A. (1971) The Hindu Dietary Practices and Culinary Rituals in a
North Indian Village, *Ethnomedizin*, **1**, 43–70.
Dumont, L. (1972) *Homo Hierarchus: The Caste System and its Implications*,
Paladin, London.

Marriott, M. (1968) Caste Ranking and Food Transactions: a Matrix Analysis, in *Structure and Change in Indian Society,* (eds M. Singer and B.S. Cohn), Aldine Publishing, Chicago.
Mayer, A.D. (1960) *Caste and Kinship in Central India: A Village and its Region,* University of California Press, Berkeley.
Kahn's account of Wamiran society is a superb example of how social dynamics are expressed, interpreted and manipulated in terms of food.
Kahn, M. (1986) *Always hungry, never greedy: Food and the expression of hunger in a Melanesian society,* Cambridge University Press, Cambridge.
For a fuller discussion of the 'bottle-babies' syndrome, see:
Jelliffe, D.B. and Jelliffe, E.F.P. (1978) *Human Milk in the Modern World,* Oxford University Press, Oxford.
Raphael, D. (1973) The Role of Breast Feeding in a Bottle Oriented World, *Ecol. Food & Nutr.,* **2,** 121–6.

DISCUSSION QUESTIONS

1. Discuss the ubiquitous spread of cola drinks in the light of status seeking.
2. Use the notions of hospitality, charity and rationing to describe systems of food sharing in your own community, region or country.
3. What local or national foods would you say have high status? Give reasons for your choices.
4. When guests bring a food or drink item with them, to what extent are they offering friendship and to what extent are they discharging a social obligation? How does this vary according to the nature of the event, e.g. potluck, formal dinner, cocktail party?
5. What variables do you think influence what people bring to a potluck meal?
6. In your culture, what foods are judged to be suitable for birthdays for (i) children and (ii) adults? Discuss the symbolic value of these foods.
7. For a chosen festival, categorize it as Ecofest, Theofest, Secular or Personal. Explore the origins and contemporary celebration of the festival noting either continuity or change in its nature and function over time.

CHAPTER 5

Food and gender

*If you're a hunter and you have some camels, the
small stock belongs to the women. If you're dairy
farmers, the chickens belong to the women. If all
you have are ducks, the ducks belong to the men.*

MEAD (1976)

SEXUAL DIVISION OF LABOUR

In widely diverse societies nearly all aspects of food-getting from production to consumption demonstrate differential gender involvement, with women usually being responsible for the greater share of food-related activities. Murdock's analysis of pre-literate societies indicated that in about three-quarters of the over 200 situations studied, cooking was exclusively a female role. In only five instances was it exclusively masculine. Hunting and fishing tended to be masculine pursuits whereas grinding grain and fetching water were predominantly women's work. Soil preparation, planting, tending and harvesting crops were less consistently allocated to one gender or the other (Murdock, 1937). This pretty well holds true today (with some notable exceptions), with the hunting and trapping of animals and birds being men's work, while women gather food, water and fuel, prepare vegetable foods and cook (Murdock and Provost, 1973). A contemporary Indian example of work differentiation based on sex is illustrated in Table 5.1.

Another clear example of strict though interdependent sexual division of labour is that of taro production by the Wamirans of Melanesia. Only Wamiran men prepare the new taro plots, working at first communally then individually. Once the plots are prepared each man then secretly plants his taro garden, using his own magic to protect it. Following planting the process of cultivation is passed to the women who work communally, digging irrigation catchment hollows around the plants and weeding. About 2 months later the women mound up earth around the plant base and cut away dried and shrivelled leaves. Then they pass the work back to their husbands for the harvesting (Kahn, 1986).

Table 5.1 Food-related sexual division of labour in Gujarat

Type of work	Women's duties	Men's duties
Domestic	Assist husband with house repairs	Occasional house repairs
	House cleaning	Look after bullocks
	Get water Cook and serve food Grind grains Tend and milk cows Wash clothes Collect fuel Child care	
Agriculture	Help cut shrubs and repair field embankments	Cut shrubs and repair field embankments
		Plough fields
	Help to sow crops	Sow crops
	Weed fields	Weed fields and irrigate crops
	Transplant seedlings	
	Harvest and thresh crop	Harvest and thresh crop
	Carry crops home	Carry crops home
		Buy inputs and market outputs

Adapted from Gopinath, C. and Kalro, A.H. (1985) India: Gujarat Medium Irrigation Project, in *Gender Roles in Development Projects*, (eds C. Overholt *et al.*), Kumarian Press, West Hartford, p. 300.

There are political and ideological consequences to assigning different productive tasks to different family members. The products of these tasks are assigned value, and their producers social worth, in ways that reinforce the social structure of the household and the power relations within it (Weismantel, 1988). In traditional Zimbabwean Ndebele society the family was a unified force where all members were interdependent and equally important in spite of the different tasks they carried out. Traditionally, women had 'life-giving' power and status in their communities. They were the ones who bore and raised children and managed the homes. They were the ones who prepared the food and without women no-one would eat. Therefore they were worthy of tremendous respect. Preparing food and managing the home was not seen as a burden but as a badge of women's power and centrality to the family

(World Food Day Association of Canada, 1993). With the development of cash economies and the commodification of food, women's role in subsistence food activities came to be devalued relative to men's role in food production for cash. As one consequence of this shift of values women's status and power within the family and socially has diminished.

Whereas anthropologists have focused mostly on traditional and developing cultures, there is evidence of similar links between food, gender and power in industrialized societies. Gussow (1986) believes that food-related activity has been divided in such a way as whatever can be translated into money and power is in the hands of men while the use of food to produce healthy human beings has been deprived of power and left to women. Thus commercial food production, food technology, and agribusiness are male dominated while feeding the family is a female role. As the science of economics developed it was (and to a large degree still is) almost exclusively concerned with measuring activity in the cash marketplace. Women's domestic role in food production and family subsistence and their role in non-cash market activity was discounted in economic reckonings and, eventually, in general social discourse.

The importance of women in food provision may be recognized when it serves the greater interest of the dominant ideology. For example, Bentley (1992) illustrates how attitudes towards women's food-related roles were manipulated in the period of food rationing in the United States during the time of the Second World War. Images of women and food were used as propaganda tools to present a reassuring picture of a stable social order despite the mayhem created by the war. Home production and consumption of food was promoted as a patriotic activity so that '...the family dinner became a weapon of war, and the kitchen a woman's battlefront'. Women were also told not to hoard rationed foods or to buy on the black-market but, at the same time, to ensure that the diets of their husbands and children were nutritionally adequate and psychologically satisfying. Gender differences were seen in meat and sugar rationing.

In the 1980s two British sociologists carried out a major study of 200 women in the Northern England city of York, gathering qualitative information about the role that food played in their lives (Kerr and Charles, 1986; Charles and Kerr, 1988). Emerging from this study were a number of insights into women and family food practices. Sexual division of labour and power relationships within the family were found to have an impact not only on actual family food consumption but also on women's ideas concerning the food needs of family members. These ideas were expressed in a differential distribution of foods between sexes and intergenerationally. Men's food needs were seen to be privileged and women cooked primarily for their husbands and children rather than for themselves. Such food privileging of men was taken for granted irrespective of need, evidence that it was based on a social ideology rather than on biological requirements.

Corroborating evidence comes from studies with French farming families where it was found that men had power, status and control over money. Women were responsible for domestic tasks and the dirtiest and most arduous farm chores, which in turn reinforced their low status. Food distribution reflected the status of family members with the male head of household and the eldest son receiving portions larger than, and of superior quality to those allocated to women, younger sons, daughters and seniors (Delphy, 1979; Delphy and Leonard, 1984). The authors conclude that the sexual division of labour and the unequal food consumption don't just justify each other, they both derive from family hierarchy. Women's experience of the sexual division of labour concerning food is well captured in a performance art piece by Sondra Segal and Roberta Sklar (Table 5.2).

FOOD-GETTING

Up until the 1970s food-getting in traditional societies was viewed in the literature primarily in terms of hunting. Man, it was assumed, was the hunter and so, ipso facto, man was the primary food provider. More recent work has made it abundantly clear that this picture is far from accurate. Firstly, women often took part in collective hunting, especially of small game and fish, and occasionally were the chief hunters. Secondly, even in hunting societies (except perhaps for in the high Arctic latitudes) the gathering of food was of prime importance and probably provided the bulk of subsistence needs. Foraging for wild foods, although carried out by both men and women, was and is a predominantly female activity.

Similarly, modern views of men as the prime agricultural producers are misleading. In Africa women are responsible for 75% of agricultural production, though only 4% are counted as economically active. African women do 30% of ploughing; 50% of planting; 50% of livestock care; 60% of harvesting; 70% of weeding; 85% of processing; 95% of domestic work (WFDAC, 1993). Women's labour is one of the factors which determine how much land can be cultivated and how well, so that the number of acres sown is more likely to be dependent on the number of females rather than males in a farming family (Rogers, 1981). Pressure on women's time is an important constraint on raising agricultural production and rural living standards. This pressure may be actually increased by technological innovations designed to increase food production. In Sierra Leone tractors and tillers were introduced to help with rice growing. This shortened the workday for the men – who were responsible for ploughing – but increased the women's workday by 50% as they were responsible for weeding and, thanks to the tractors, now had larger areas of land to weed (WFDAC, 1993). In Java, socioeconomic and technological changes have contributed to decreased employment opportunities for

Food and gender

Table 5.2 The Hunter, the Gatherer, the Shopper, the Cook*

But I've been cooking all day.
Standing over a hot stove.
Slaving over a hot stove.
Cooking.
I've been shopping for groceries.
Putting them away.
Setting the table.
Cooking the food.
Making this dinner.
Wracking my brains.
I've been wracking my brains over this meal.
What to buy.
How much to pay.
I've been budgeting.
Looking for sales.
I've been feeding this family on $6.00.
Making it do.
I've been wracking my brains over this meal.

I have been cooking all day.
Shopping for bargains.
Hunting for bargains.
I've been hunting all day.
I've been up and down hundreds of aisles.
Hunting.
Hunting and gathering and cooking this food.
Loading my cart.
Carrying carcasses.
I have been hunting all day.
I have gathered this food from across the land.
I've been everywhere.
I've been everywhere.
I have made this meal.
I have created this food.
This is my time.
My thought.
What you have on your plate is my blood.
My brains.
I tell you I have been cooking all day.

What do you mean
    you don't want it?

---

* From *Woman's Body & Other Natual Resources*, by Sondra Segal and Roberta Sklar (1987).

women in agriculture. The rising price of rice led to a shift from communal planting and harvesting, where crops are shared to single family enterprises where the crop is sold. The light hand-held knives traditionally used for harvesting have been replaced by heavier steel sickles, which can only be wielded by men. This has drastically changed labour patterns, reducing 200 women-days of harvest work to 70 men-days. Similarly, rotary weeders – again used only by men – are replacing hand weeding by women and reducing 20 women-days of work to 8 men-days (Pyle, 1985).

Women, who in the developing world produce over 50% of the world's food, have little control over land and resources, receive little recognition or assistance in food production, and are generally invisible to policy makers, credit institutions and urban consumers (Sivard, 1985). It is the man who drives the tractor or who sows the cash crops and so it is the man who receives inputs of money, credit, tools and advice in the name of improving productivity.

In Africa, colonial taxation policies often forced men into wage labour on plantations or in industries thus integrating them into the cash-based economy. This mass migration of male labour left women responsible for household food production and subsistence agriculture. Today, in Lesotho 50% of rural women farm alone because their husbands are working in neighbouring South Africa (Twose, 1987). Wages from men's work are often insufficient to feed their families or are spent on luxuries rather than food. Among the Ecuadorians of Zumbagua, men work in the city of Quito, only returning to the village at times of peak agricultural activity and when wives are about to give birth. This leaves women to do all the food and subsistence tasks. Pasturing sheep is normally done by older children; when they go to school, women have to do this too. Men return from work, often with food gifts of candy rather than the rice and flour which is needed. This division of households into proletarian males and subsidence-farmer females permits the transfer of value from the rural to capitalist sector but does little to benefit the family either materially or socially (Weismantel, 1988).

Similar processes can be seen to be at work in Canada. After colonization vast amounts of land were converted to wheat production for export. The financial success of early ventures was dependent on the labour of farm women who grew vegetables, raised poultry, preserved food for the winters and largely bore the responsibility of feeding the family. Today in Canada, men and women farmers often have off-farm jobs to make ends meet, and many family farms survive only because of the unpaid agricultural and subsistence labour of women.

FOOD PREPARATION

Food preparation is part of that non-economic sector of activities which is nevertheless crucial to the existence and expansion of the economic sector. In subsistence situations it takes an enormous amount of work after the harvest is in to produce food in an edible form; in fact the time required to prepare a staple may exceed the time to cultivate it in the first place. There are several time–budget studies on food-related activities (especially in Asia) showing that women have longer and harder tasks related to food preparation than do men. Threshing, winnowing, drying, boiling and other activities have to be undertaken between the harvesting and storing of many staple foods. As the food is used, more work is involved in processing it (stamping of grains, grinding, husking, extraction of toxins; e.g. from cassava). Before cooking, an adequate supply of water and fuel needs to be obtained. Cooking itself takes considerable time, especially if fuel sources need to be conserved. Relishes, vegetables or spices needed to make food palatable have to be gathered separately or cultivated. All are essential tasks, performed by women (Rogers, 1981). The demands of post-harvest preparation place major constraints on food production and may be a factor inducing people to switch to foods requiring less processing or to ready-processed foods, with the nutritional and economic consequences that entails. Describing life in Zumbagua, Ecuador, Weismantel (1988) says that women get up early to start grinding and toasting barley, while men stay in bed waiting to be served hot water and m chica (a grain drink). In a large household one woman does the first grinding, another woman the second fine grinding and sifting, and senior women toast the grain, boil the water and fill the bowls, handing them to a young grand-daughter to carry to the men. A woman who runs a kitchen by herself with only children to help must grind barley the day before.

In industrialized countries, where ready-processed foods are the norm, food procurement mostly involves shopping at commercial stores and supermarkets, whereas preparation is restricted to relatively simple and less labour intensive operations like peeling, chopping and mixing. Most often, women are responsible for these tasks and it may be thought therefore that they control what food ends up on the family table. However, women in Kerr and Charles' study of British families reported that to cater for each family member's preferences was expensive as well time consuming and for that reason it was easier to plan meals around their husband's preferences. Women's knowledge of their partner's food preferences is derived by trial and error in the early stages of their relationship. Women report feelings of guilt, concern or unworthiness when the food they have prepared is rejected and are unlikely to repeat such a 'mistake', while at the same time they subordinate or even deny their own food preferences.

Men may also indirectly influence food selection by controlling the amount of money budgeted for food and thereby setting limits to the quantity and quality and type of food purchased. 'I send him out at the end of the month cos he'll buy extras on top of the budget – which I'd never do 'cos he'd go mad and say I wasn't managing properly'

(Calnan and Fieldhouse, 1986). Eisenbraun (1987) comments that in effect men have undermined women's roles as gatekeepers, dictating by their preferences what food will be purchased and prepared. It is evident of course that women do make decisions about food procurement and preparation, but this may be in the nature of what Safilios-Rothschild (1970) calls implementation power. Such power is subordinate to orchestration power which is the power to make important and infrequent decisions which determine the lifestyle of the family. An individual with orchestration power also has the power to delegate unimportant and time-consuming decisions to their spouse, who thus acquires implementation power. So in our example, women get delegated the food shopping, but they don't necessarily control what is bought.

COOKING

Cooking is usually a female task though it is an area where sexual division of labour may be flexible. For example, Zumbaguan men will cook while their wives are in childbirth and Bemba men take over cooking and other women's tasks when chiefs require tributary labour. In the West, men may cook when forced to by a woman's illness or absence. (Their supposed, or expected, inability to do so has provided the basis for many jokes and situation comedies.) As has been remarked elsewhere, when men cook it is more likely to be for a special occasion or to involve prestige foods, while women still do the everyday cooking. All over India, ceremonial food is cooked by men. (An interesting gender distinction is seen with Sushi, which is made only by men as it is thought that only cool male hands are of the right temperature to shape the sticky rice.)

Although women do the cooking, what is cooked may be circumscribed by men's preferences. The idea of a 'proper meal' is a strong one in traditional British working-class families. The proper meal is defined as 'meat-and-two-veg', with gravy as a unifying element and it is both highly valued and a yardstick by which other meals are judged. This limits the scope for innovation. 'It's the same every week you know, he's not a one for fancy cooking at all. If I put a lasagne in front of him he'd throw it at me, y'know. He likes pork chops, chicken and fish, and that usually makes the seven days up.' (Kerr and Charles, 1986). The preparation of a proper meal symbolizes the woman's role as homemaker by ensuring that she has been in the kitchen for a given period of time before her husband returns home (Murcott, 1982). In this way women's place in the home is confirmed and social expectations fulfilled.

Gussow (1988) notes that getting women out of the kitchen has been a goal of 'everyone from Lenin to the N.O.W.' (National

Organization of Women), and that cooking is generally regarded as being regressive. However she also points out that there is no evidence that women hated cooking to begin with. In fact, in industrialized countries there is relatively little information on women's attitudes toward food preparation or on their cooking skills. Some sociological studies in the 1970s and 1980s suggested that cooking is among the most liked of household tasks although women get tired of inventing new dishes and washing up afterwards. Oakley (1974) criticizes women's magazines for encouraging the illusion that cooking is a creative pleasure when in fact it should be classed as work – work which is neither recognized as such nor paid. This is certainly the case made for developing countries, above. However, does the perspective change in a non-subsistence situation? Although cooking in the home has parallels to paid work in that it is usually not a matter of choice and it is governed by social expectations and constraints, it can undoubtedly also be a pleasure, or indeed a hobby. Mennel (1985) suggests that there is a middle category between work and pleasure which can be termed 'private work and family management' into which cooking falls. Through a study of English women's magazines he shows how utilitarian attitudes toward food gave way after the Second World War to a view of cooking as a source of enjoyment and adventure, of achievement and social status; and how start-from-scratch recipes now alternate with those which 'take the most ruthless short cuts with convenience foods'. While it is obviously true that cooking can be an intrinsically rewarding activity, the concept of private work and family management may be yet another way of avoiding recognition of the economic value of women's work.

The liberation of women from the kitchen was also a promise of the manufacturers of kitchen gadgets and convenience foods. However, as Gussow (1987) shows, there is little evidence that this was ever the real intention and certainly not the outcome. Food industry supporters argue that convenience foods were a response to the needs of women who wanted to get out of the home. Critics suggest that industry advertising deliberately depicted cookery as time-consuming drudgery in order to create a market for its goods. Certainly, the time women spend on food preparation has changed little in 50 years. Gussow also discusses the issue of whether home cooking is an economically sound behaviour, concluding that for the simplest canned and frozen foods and most highly paid women, cooking may not always pay, but for most foods and most women it probably does. So in moving out of the home in order to gain the status of participating in the formal economic sector, women have saved neither time nor money spent on food and may have given up something which was a source of satisfaction.

FOOD SERVING

When a woman serves a dish she has prepared, this offering of her labour for another's consumption is intrinsically an act of subordination. Moreover, it is a cross-culturally common symbol.

Weismantel (1988)

The rituals and mechanics of serving food continue to emphasize differences between gender roles and status. Porotas Granados a la Chilena is a celebratory harvest dish eaten by many Chileans. The woman prepares the meal with help of older daughters and does not eat until everyone else has finished. Among the nomadic Gadulia Lohars of Northern India food is served first to the men and children, then the women eat whatever remains. In Gitksan society, men were always served before women and children. If there were guests the women of the household did not sit down to eat but tended to the needs of the visitors. Weismantel (1988) describes the serving of meals at harvest time in Ecuador. Seating follows a hierarchy based on old before young, male before female, guest before host. As a rule men sit above the ground while women sit on it. (For ordinary family meals this seating hierarchy is dispensed with.) The senior woman of the house remains seated by the fire, ladling food into bowls, while a child or younger woman serves it. The older woman, being in absolute control of the process, has three powerful devices to employ to express messages about social status and power and perhaps to challenge the status quo. First of all she controls the order of serving; as she ladles each portion she indicates for whom it is intended. She also has at her disposal bowls and spoons of different sizes, shapes, designs and materials. The biggest, newest and most ornate goes to the person first served thus reinforcing the status distinction already expressed by the serving order. To some extent it is pragmatic; children get the smallest least fragile bowls; men who do heaviest work get the biggest portions. By introducing incongruities between serving order and serving size, the woman can express subtle social distinctions and favouritisms. The third aspect of her control lies in deciding the composition of each serving of soup. Meat and potatoes, set aside in separate dishes, are added to the broth at the time of serving in amounts calculated to be appropriate to social status. Each diner must thank the server both on receiving the full bowl and returning it empty and cannot refuse if enjoined to 'please eat more'. The server role as a symbol of women's subordination 'provides the woman who wields the ladle the chance to smugly hand out excruciating insults while meekly proclaiming her utter lack of political power'. The meal thus represents the subordination of female to male and yet is a locus of feminine power within the family.

FOOD CONSUMPTION

It has long been recognized as a home-truth that when food is scarce women often do without, to the detriment of their health and strength, in order to ensure that their children receive adequate nourishment. Such behaviour has been documented in case studies of families with very low incomes in regions as diverse as Morocco, India and Central America (Bhatty, 1980; Maher, 1984; Menchu, 1985). Historically, instances of maternal self-sacrifice have been recorded in accounts of Canadian home-steaders as well as among the British working classes. Although patterns of food distribution in families under the stressful conditions imposed by food shortages have been well studied, systematic investigations of what might be called ordinary non-crisis conditions is limited.

Generally, from a simple physiological perspective, men have higher nutritional requirements than women, and this fact must not be ignored when examining the gender basis of food consumption. However, it does not necessarily hold true in individual circumstances. Rogers (1981) notes that in the developing world although women who are lactating or pregnant and doing very heavy farm work may need the same or more calories than men, often the men have first choice of the families' food and they have the most of the available cash with which to buy extra food and drinks. In Zumbagua, men are served more meat than women, and older adults before younger ones. Nonetheless, distribution of protein by gender may actually favour women despite appearances to the contrary, because women frequently cook themselves titbits of meat while making a meal (Weismantel, 1988).

Table 5.3 The Hierarchy of the Chicken

The father eats the breast.
He only likes white meat.
The kids eat the drumsticks,
    the thighs, and
    the wings.
The mother eats the neck
    the back
    the liver
    the gizzard
    the feet
    and the heart.

---

* From *Woman's Body & Other Natural Resources*, by Sondra Segal and Roberta Sklar (1987).

In Westernized settings, men serve themselves first in family-style service where bowls of food are placed on the table and from which everyone helps themselves. With plated meals men get choicer pieces and larger portions regardless of actual physiological need (Table 5.3). Although some women recognize this biological inequity, they also talk of deserving less. '... if I put it on the plate and I suddenly think there's quite a lot on my plate I always take it off because I feel guilty. But I pile it on his plate. I do sometimes, I think I could eat the amount he has and he could eat the amount I have quite happily.' (Kerr and Charles, 1986). The extent to which women internalize the belief that men deserve to be privileged with respect to food consumption is seen to be illustrative of their subordination in the household. Eisenbraun (1987) provides a summary and a critique of the privileging thesis which also draws attention to problems in interpretation of findings.

SUMMARY

In most societies, the position of women in terms of equity, economic opportunities and rewards is different from and inferior to that of men. Food-related activities take place in the context of these unequal social and material relationships, reproducing and perpetuating the asymmetry.

For educators and advertisers alike women are perceived to be the major agents of change for food habits within households. This general supposition reflects the notion of the housewife as a gatekeeper, controlling the flow of food into the household. Analyses such as those of Kerr and Charles challenge this supposition and instead describe the role of women as being that of servers whose needs are subordinated to male preferences and requirements. 'The preparation of food is considered an act of servitude, the demonstration of a subordinate and servicing social position.... The meal is the product of woman's domestic labor, demonstrating her willingness to serve the family' (Coward, 1985).

Dahlberg (1981) notes that there is a heterogeneity in food-getting strategies of diverse peoples throughout history that precludes any easy generalizations being made about the role and status of women. For example, theories that base women's status on primary food production alone do not explain the fact that Chipewyan women possess inherent power despite being totally dependent on men for food procurement. She says that the evidence shows flexibility in roles and beliefs resulting in interdependence and cooperation between men and women.

The views of women as gatekeepers to family food or as mere servers of men's needs are both open to challenge. Food-related activities are part of a negotiated contract, the rules of which are sometimes explicit but more often implicitly understood. Nevertheless, to the extent that family food choices do occur within a social ideological framework then it is clear that nutrition education strategies which focus on individual behaviour change will not be adequate. No amount of sound advice will be helpful if recommended changes, aimed primarily at women, conflict with either ideological or material realities. More attention must be given to influencing the nature of the overall food supply and to influencing the cost, social status and acceptability of nutritionally desirable foods, so that easy choices are healthy choices are culturally acceptable choices.

FURTHER READING

Dahlberg, F. (1981) *Woman the Gatherer*, Yale University Press, New Haven. An introduction to women as hunters and gatherers, with contributed case studies from around the world illustrating differing food-related gender roles.

Charles, N. and Kerr, M. (1988) *Women, Food and Families*, Manchester University Press, Manchester. A detailed account of the study of 200 British women and family food, including numerous passages in the women's own words.

Weismantel, M.J. (1988) *Food, Gender and Poverty in the Ecuadorian Andes*, University of Pennsylvania Press, Philadelphia. An ethnographic study focusing on food and cooking. Full of useful information and insights on biocultural uses and meanings of food.

World Food Day Association of Canada (1993) *The Hand That Feeds the World: Women's Role in Global Food Security*, Ottawa, The Author. This is a curriculum resource kit comprising video and printed guide, which investigates the links between gender issues, food security, agribusiness and environmental issues.

Overholt, C., Anderson, M.B., Cloud, K. and Austin, J.E. (eds) (1985) *Gender Roles in Development Projects: A Case Book*, Kumarian Press, West Hartford. A collection of papers examining the role of women in development projects, including agricultural and nutritional perspectives.

DISCUSSION QUESTIONS

1. Does the analysis bought to bear on food and power for British women hold in other situations and other cultures? Discuss this in the context of any or all of the following; fast-food culture; the trend to eating out; changing family structures; changing family lifestyles.
2. An extraordinary amount of female time and energy is devoted to dieting, reading about dieting and working out. Discuss the proposition that women spend more time now avoiding food than they once did obtaining it.
3. Why do you think that the time that women spend on food preparation has not substantially changed in the last 50 years?

4. Discuss the importance of women's work in the context of food security, at a household, community, regional or national level.
5. Describe gender differences in food-related activities in a selected cultural group.
6. Can male privileging with respect to meat be adequately explained as a legacy of hunter societies?

CHAPTER 6

Religion

Religion is fundamentally a belief system which includes the myths that explain the social and religious order and the rituals through which the members of the religious community carry out their beliefs and act out the myths to explain the unknown (Freidl and Pfeiffer, 1977). Its purpose is to express beliefs about the Universe and to fulfil a basic need by helping people to cope with the unknown and uncontrollable. World religions may be divided broadly into two types; prophetic and mystical. Prophetic religions are derived from ancient Jewish lore and include also Christianity and Islam. The mystical religions originate in Indian philosophies; they are sometimes classed as 'Eastern'. Under this division Islam is properly classed as a 'Western' religion. Each religion has its own rituals and ceremonies; its own special beliefs; its own interpretation of morality. The practices of religious adherents are an attempt by them to relate to the supreme being they worship; to explain those things which they themselves cannot fully understand or control, and adherence to religious laws is important in reaffirming the beliefs of that religion (Brown, 1963).

THE FUNCTION OF RELIGIOUS FOOD PRACTICES

Religious adherents around the world are more or less circumscribed in their food choices by the teachings of their chosen faith. Religious food symbolism is common, and many religious rituals involve food. The specifics vary, of course, but the nature and function of food practices is similar in all religions; they fall into one or more of six general functional categories.

1. Communication with God or other supernatural forces
2. Demonstration of faith
3. Rejection of worldliness
4. Enhancement of feelings of identity or belongingness
5. Expression of separateness
6. Reinforcement of ecological pragmatism

Communicating with supernatural forces

Sacrifices to gods are common ways of trying to avoid undesirable events or of ensuring favourable events. They may be in the nature of supplications, for example to ensure favourable conditions for Spring planting, or appeasements, as in thanksgiving for a bountiful harvest. Sacrifices, which were once human in nature have given way to animal or plant sacrifices or to purely symbolic acts. Thus the giving up of certain foods for Lent may be seen to be a sacrifice just as much as is the slaughter of a goat, or plant offerings at Harvest Festivals. Sacrificial meals allow people to gather together to eat foods which have been offered to the gods and which are then eaten in their presence. They thus serve the function of creating both religious and secular bonds.

The gods themselves may be the meal. Just as ancient theories of correspondence suggested that the hunter who ate the heart of a leopard would acquire the beast's bravery, symbolically eating the god allows the eater to acquire godly virtues, or at the least to identify spiritually with the god. The case of the Eucharist, already discussed in Chapter 4, is examined from another angle later in the section on Christianity.

Demonstrating faith

Symbolic remembrance of historical events is a way of constantly reaffirming, privately and publically, one's faith. Asarah-Be-Tebeth is one of four fast days commemorating the siege and fall of Jerusalem under Nebuchadnezzar (Table 6.1), whereas Sukkot, or the festival of the Tabernacles commemorates the wanderings of the Israelites in the desert after the exodus from Egypt. Unquestioning obedience to dietary laws also demonstrates full acceptance of religious authority. For Observant Jews no rational explanation of their complex dietary regulations is required; it is enough that the laws are the word of God.

Table 6.1 Jewish fast days commemorating the siege and fall of Jerusalem

Fast of the tenth month (10th of Tebeth)	Commencement of siege
Fast of the fourth month (17th of Tammuz)	First breach of the walls
Fast of the fifth month (9th of Ab)	Destruction of temple
Fast of the seventh month (3rd of Tishri)	Assassination of Gedahiah, governor of Judah

Rejecting worldliness

Self-denial is highly valued or promoted in many religious codes. The rejection of worldly desires may be shown by unconcern for ways of the flesh – including eating. Fasting in one form or another is an almost universal practice and fasts are very common events in religious calendars. Fasts are undertaken in preparation for important religious events or as acts of penance, remembrance or of supplication. Fasting is a way to free the soul from pre-occupation with worldly matters so that one is spiritually prepared to commune with God. Frequently, the general populace observes only special fast days whereas more ascetic adherents will forego food on a regular basis. In some instances holy men and women will fast on behalf of the general population.

Enhancing identity and belongingness

Individuals who observe codified food rules make a public demonstration of belonging to a group, and every day provide themselves with a private affirmation of identification with the group. In this way sense of belonging is constantly reinforced. Indeed, some religious food practices may have been decreed expressly to create such a feeling of fellowship and group membership. In obeying the dietary laws one is continually reminded that one is a member of the Faith. The need to preserve identity is especially felt when one group is threatened by assimilation into a larger or more powerful group. At one time Jews were forbidden to drink wine with non-Jews as a means of restricting social intercourse which might have led to intermarriage with gentiles and ultimately to cultural assimilation. Eating together, which is often an integral part of religious ceremonies, contributes to feelings of social cohesion. A funeral meal is a way of appeasing grief by reinforcing bonds that unite the living. More joyous everyday examples include church basement suppers and Sunday school picnics.

Expressing separateness

Food rules and practices may also serve to demarcate religious, social and political boundaries. Within the Hindu religion the caste system imposes rules of what may be eaten with and by whom. High-caste Brahmins may eat only 'pure' food, and thus cannot eat with or accept food from lower castes. The Mohammedan prohibition against pork is thought by some to have served the function of reminding Moslems that they were different from (and superior to) their Christian neighbours. In the eighth century CE Pope Gregory III prohibited horseflesh to Christians and Christian converts to set them apart from the horse-eating Vandals of northern Europe.

Reinforcing ecological pragmatism

Religious practices may serve, incidentally or purposefully, to encourage environmental adaptation through conservation of scarce resources and of human effort. Pig-raising, which made sense in the original forests of the Middle East uplands, gradually lost its utility as agriculture spread and the forests gave way to grasslands and eventually to desert. The new herders and farmers who replaced the nomads had to devote more of their own resources to feeding pigs who could no longer forage for themselves. A religiously sanctioned prohibition would thus serve to discourage a costly and ecologically maladaptive practice.

THE NATURE OF RELIGIOUS FOOD PRACTICES

Food practices which fulfil the functions outlined above may be characterized as either prohibiting or requiring the use of specific foods in specific situations. Some of these rules apply to everyday eating; others are concerned with special celebrations, frequently involving feasts or fasts (Table 6.2). Many foods have a powerful symbolic value.

Taboos are ways of maintaining the status quo in a group by identifying, through means of symbols, cultural rules which cannot be transgressed without danger to the individual or the group. Foods readily lend themselves to this symbolic role and cultural foodways are rich in examples of foods which are not allowed for consumption though they be freely available. What must not be eaten may be circumscribed by characteristics of individuals such as age, gender, social or physiological status, or by external constraints such as time of day or of year.

Prohibitions may be circumvented in a number of ways. One of these involves renaming the prohibited food to identify it with one which is permitted. Thus in Medieval Japan, where the advent of Buddhism resulted in a prohibition on meat eating, deer became known as Mountain Whale. Whale was considered to be a fish, and Buddhism offered no objection to eating fish. Such circumventions may be tacitly agreed upon as being necessary for survival, especially if the prohibited food is an essential food source in times of scarcity. The Hindu prohibition on slaughtering cows may be circumvented by allowing Moslem butchers to do the bloody deed. Jews place health above the strictures of dietary laws.

Prescriptive rules of what must be eaten, when and how, are the counterpart of prohibitions. For example, on the eve of the Jewish festival of Yom Kippur, meat-filled dumplings known as kreplach should be eaten. The Moslem Ramadhan fast has to be broken as soon after sunset each day as possible. Traditionally among Moslems, only the right hand should be used for eating with, as the left hand is considered to be unclean. Prescriptive rules though, are most often associated with specific ceremonies or rituals where particular foods have acquired symbolic meanings. For example, in Greek Orthodox practice, boiled bulgar wheat known as kolyva or koljivo is used as a symbol of everlasting life. Mixed with pomegranate seeds, nuts and spices, it is offered at the altar 3, 9 and

Table 6.2 Comparative examples of religious dietary strictures

Food restrictions		
	Judaism	● Eat only animals with cloven hooves and which chew the cud, ie. cattle, sheep, goats, deer ● Eat only forequarters of animal ● Eat only fish with scales and fins ● No blood
	Islam	● No blood ● No pork ● No intoxicating liquor
	Sikhism	● No beef
	Hinduism	● Must not kill or eat any animal
Days of the year		
	Christianity	● No meat on Fridays during Lent (Catholics) ● Fast Wednesday and Friday (Greek Orthodox) (with the exception of two weeks) ● No food preparation on Sabbath (Mormons, Seventh Day Adventists)
	Judaism	● No food preparation on Sabbath
Time of day		
	Islam	● Foods may not be eaten between sunrise and sunset during Ramadhan
	Buddhism	● Monks do not eat after midday
Preparation of food		
	Judaism	● Ritual slaughtering of animals ● Separate utensils for meat and dairy products
	Islam	● Ritual animal slaughter
	Hinduism	● Ritual bathing and donning of clean clothes by Brahmins before eating
Fasts		
	Christian	● 40-day Great Lent fast before Easter and a 40-day Advent fast (Greek Orthodox)
	Islam	● Month of Ramadhan 13th, 14th, 15th of each month

40 days after a family death – recalling the times that Christ appeared on earth after his crucifixion. The mixture is sprinkled with sugar, as a wish that the dead will find sweetness and peace in heaven. In some countries it is also made on patron saints' days.

Fasts may vary from a few hours to many days, during which time restriction of food intake may be slight or extensive. A fast may mean forgoing only certain categories of food or it may mean complete denial of food except, perhaps, for water. Fasting may be required during the daylight hours as in the Moslem festival of Ramadhan, where it is complemented with feasting at night. Or it may occur on selected days of the week as in the Catholic practice of substituting fish for meat on Fridays.

The celebration of significant religious events typically involves using special foods or preparation methods which are usually more elaborate than everyday fare. The time and effort to prepare for such events is an indication of their importance as much as are the actual foods served.

ORIGINS OF RELIGIOUS FOOD PRACTICES

Religious food customs originate in three main ways. Some are required by the God and are described in scriptures; others are decreed by religious or political leaders; still others arise through adaptation or co-option of existing food practices for religious purposes. The Jewish Torah, the Moslem Qur'an and the Hindu Code of Manu all contain specific directives concerning food practices. Rabbis added to the Jewish dietary laws, and made interpretations where biblical direction was unclear. Pagan festivals were frequently assimilated and given new meanings as modern religions assumed dominance over older forms of worship.

A good example of this latter process is provided by the Jewish Spring festival of Passover, or Pesach, which commemorates events during the Exodus from Egypt but which is actually an amalgamation of two older pagan festivals. Hag ha-Pesah, or the Festival of the Shepherds, involved sacrifice of a Paschal lamb, the blood of which was smeared on tents to ward off misfortune. (When the Angel of Death slew the Egyptian firstborn, the Jews – who were to be spared – identified their houses by marking their doors with the blood of sacrificed animals.) The second festival was Hag ha-Matsot, an agricultural celebration marking the beginning of the Spring harvest. The first grain was baked into unleavened cakes in a ceremony of thanksgiving for the harvest. In the context of Passover, old customs were re-interpreted; matsos became the bread of affliction – symbols of oppression.

Although dietary regulations are obeyed because they are written down in Holy Books their origin may be related to particular environmental and cultural conditions. Practical advantages offered by certain food practices may have been imbued with religious virtues in order to ensure their continued practice. Many of the food prohibitions of the various religions involve meat. Simoons (1961) deals with the widespread rejection of the pig as food, noting that the Middle East is a centre of pork avoidance, where Christians and pagans, as well as Moslems and Jews, all reject pork as food. He suggests that among the pastoralists of Asia the pig was not a commonly eaten food but that it was eaten by those who settled permanently in the area. The taboo arose as an expression of contempt by one group for the other and the consequent ridiculing of each other's customs. There are many examples in food lore which show the use of food as a means to demonstrate differences between groups at society and at sub-group level. Once the prejudice against eating pork was established it could have been incorporated into religious writings as a means of accentuating and perpetuating the cultural division.

As described above it has been proposed that ecological imperatives requiring conservation of resources and thus appropriate use of land and resources was an important reason for nomads to forsake the keeping of pigs. Political motives may be seen in the control of resources as a means of ensuring obedience to authorities. Historically, Middle East rulers saw the raising of pigs as being too profitable for the villages, making them dangerously autonomous. Rulers prohibited pig rearing to prevent this threat to their power (Diener and Robkin, 1978). Practical concerns with health may also be an influencing factor. The particular case of trichinosis in pork is often cited as a reason for the forbidden status of pigs. Pork is easily infected with the parasite *Trichinella spirella* and is thus a source of disease in humans. However, such an explanation assumes a modern scientific understanding of disease processes and neglects the fact that other meats would have been equally subject to spoilage and therefore also be potential disease carrying agents.

Grivetti and Pangborn (1974) also challenge the contention that Semitic avoidance of pork is based on health and sanitation and propose instead that it involved ecological factors and the retention of ethnic identity. The Jews may have prohibited it to set themselves apart; however, this does not explain why a prohibition was placed particularly on pork. Other types of meat were eaten in common by the different cultural groups in the area and other cultural practices were also similar. Additionally, the Jewish prohibition against pork is not recorded in the Bible until after the Exodus from Egypt. Until then, every living thing was considered to be suitable food for consumption: 'Every moving thing that liveth shall be meat for you' (Genesis 9:3). Farb and Armelagos (1980) are of the opinion that the taboo can be solely explained by the Prophetic admonitions to avoid imperfection. The book of Leviticus is concerned with themes of wholeness and perfection; only that which is blessed as being perfect is acceptable to God. Such animals were those that were already domesti-cated when the Israelites first inhabited the Holy Lands (Douglas, 1970). The pig was thus excluded, together with other 'imperfect' creatures such as shellfish, rodents and lizards, insects and flightless birds. These were considered to be abominations which did not conform to what was expected of their class of living beings. Farb points out that the biblical prohibition against the pig is no more prominent than that against other imperfect animals and asks why then the pig taboo has come to be almost symbolic of Jewish diets. In the second century BCE (Before Common Era) Antiochus IV desecrated the Temple of Solomon and ordered that swine were to be sacrificed there and that Jews were to eat the meat as an act of submission to the Syrians. This gave prominence to what had been only one of a number of dietary taboos. The Hellenistic world was outraged at the enormity of this act which involved the deliberate pollution of a place of worship, and in self-defence Antiochus was forced to spread a story that Jews were in the habit of fattening up Greek prisoners, sacrificing them, and eating them while swearing hostility to the Greeks (Tannahill, 1976). When the Macabees captured Jerusalem and re-established the Temple, pork avoidance became an assertion of opposition to Pagan rule – a declaration of allegiance to the ancient Law of Moses.

The ecological explanation has been mentioned earlier. The Biblical prohibition, says Harris (1977), helped to remove any temptation to raise pigs. The other forbidden species were similarly proscribed because of the disproportionate amount of time and effort that would have had to have been expended in hunting. Thus there is a general rationale of banning inconvenient and expensive foods.

The prohibition on mixing meat and milk, referred to earlier, is widely identified as a specific Jewish practice. However, Grivetti (1980) points out that the meat/milk separation is also observed in parts of South-West Asia, Central Sahara, East Africa and South-West Africa, and that its origin in Jewish lore is therefore questionable. In the Old Testament books of Leviticus and Deuteronomy, where many of the Jewish dietary laws are set down, there is no prohibition placed on the mixing of milk and meat products; indeed such a combination is seen to be of high status. It is the commandment against seething, found in Exodus, which is the basis for the prohibition. Grivetti pursues this discrepancy and reviews evidence for a number of possible origins for the practice, of which the biblical commandment is only one. Hypotheses include notions of health and of ethnic identity, which we have already encountered in relation to pork; the idea of self-denial (undue pleasure is gained from eating both foods); conservation of staples (protein foods were too precious to be used unsparingly); and sympathetic magic. In regard to the latter Grivetti says that African pastoralists do not boil milk as they believe that this will prevent further milk production from that cow; boiling a kid in its mother's milk would therefore represent a threat to the whole herd. Some scholars have suggested that the problem rests on the mistranslation of 'blood' as 'milk' in the Biblical injunction. Grivetti finds little to commend this idea but instead favours an explanation based on semantic manipulation. The Biblical text, he says, referred to the preparation of food rather than to the consumption of it. It did not forbid the mixing of milk and meat at the same meal, but only during preparation of the meal; modern Orthodox practice is thus based on a misunderstanding. Examples such as this illustrate the difficulty in determining the origin of food practices and also the ease with which later rationalizations become established and are accepted as true explanations.

Even if prohibitions arise for sound ecological or cultural reasons there is still the question of why they persist when conditions change. It may become obvious that the breaking of a particular food law does not have any adverse consequences, in which case prohibitions may indeed be lifted. However, if the consequences, real or imagined, are severe enough then the prohibition will persist. The social sanctions against eating forbidden foods may be strong enough to cause fear and guilt sufficient to deter anyone from even trying them. This fear may cause actual physical symptoms; thus the very thought of eating pork is enough to make an Orthodox Jew feel physically sick. Those who do dare to break the taboo may also suffer symptoms of physical sickness induced, perhaps psychosomatically, by the expectation of a negative reaction to the eating of forbidden foods. This is in the nature of a self-fulfilling prophecy, and those who survive such distressing experiences are unlikely to ever touch the food again (Farb and Armelagos, 1980).

THE CHANGING NATURE OF RELIGIOUS FOOD PRACTICES

Like any foodways, religious food practices are dynamic; they are subject to continuous change and adaptation. Changes may occur as result of religious reform or revisionism, acculturation, individual, family or community adaptations.

Adherence to dietary laws or guidelines varies between and within religious groups on a national, regional, community, family or individual level. In many cases religions have developed several branches, sects or schools of thought which make different demands on members. A good example is provided by Judaism. Orthodox and Conservative Jews follow similar standards of Kashruth based on biblical, rabbinic and customary rules. Conservatives tend to follow more lenient options within the law. Reform Jews do not regard Kashruth as binding.

Individuals and families may adapt and vary traditional practices to suit personal needs and preferences or to reflect new family traditions. An example of change in what would appear to be a static religious food event is provided by Sherman's ethnographic account of seder celebrations in one family. This illustrates how families can adapt a traditional and important religious ceremony by incorporating local customs and food preferences while retaining its underlying form and meaning (Sherman, 1991).

Immigration provides a good example of how changing circumstances may result in changing attitudes to dietary practices. Through the process of acculturation dietary practices are modified in the light of availability of foodstuffs and as an adaptation to new cultural rules, customs and expectations. Compliance may also depend on social contexts. Adherents who are strict when with members of their own religious group may be willing to be more lax when alone or with a different social group. Influences which come into play include freedom from peer pressure to conform, and deference to a host's dietary practices.

FOOD BELIEFS AND PRACTICES IN WORLD RELIGIONS

Christianity

Christianity comprises three main groups, Roman Catholic, Protestant and Eastern Orthodox, including numerous sects and non-conformists. The saying of a short prayer before and after eating, establishing a direct connection between God and good food, is common among Christian groups. Other than this, dietary strictures differ between groups, being almost non-existent in the Protestant and Catholic Churches and quite strict in the Eastern Orthodox Church.

Until 1966, Roman Catholics were required to abstain from eating meat on Fridays (since applied only to Fridays during Lent) in symbolic remembrance of the death of Christ. The historic consequence of meat avoidance on Fridays was the regular consumption of fish; fish Fridays became identified with Roman Catholicism and so fish was deliberately avoided by some other Christian sects who did not wish to be mistaken for Catholics.

The first disciples of Jesus observed Mosaic laws. However, with the spread of Christianity across cultural as well as geographical boundaries these practices became increasingly irrelevant and, except in the Eastern Orthodox Church, most Christian dietary laws had disappeared by the end of the second century CE. It was not until much later that Protestant sects such as the Seventh Day Adventists and the Mormons established dietary rules anew.

Seventh Day Adventism

Officially organized in 1863, the Seventh Day Adventists are a religious sect whose main tenet of Faith is that the second coming of Christ on earth is imminent. As in Judaism, the Sabbath is a day of rest, and no food may be prepared on that day. Instead, food may be readied on Friday and the dishes washed on Sunday.

Much emphasis is placed on healthful living achieved by eating the right foods and taking exercise and rest. 'Surely you know that you are God's temple, where the Spirit of God dwells. Anyone who destroys God's temple will himself be destroyed by God, because the temple of God is holy; and that temple you are.' (1 Corinthians 3:16–17). Probably about half of Adventists are vegetarians, the majority of these being lacto-ovo vegetarians. Meat is rejected for several reasons including biblical

references to uncleanliness of swine. Mrs Ellen White, an early and influential convert to Adventism, held that meat consumption made people
animalistic and unsympathetic to others. Non-vegetarian Adventists
usually eat meat in smaller than average quantities. Lacto-ovo vegetarian
menus are the norm for Adventist schools and hospitals, though the latter
are increasingly serving non-vegetarian diets to patients (Bosley and
Hardinge, 1992). Tea, coffee, alcohol and tobacco are also avoided, and
the use of hot spices and aged cheeses is discouraged. Eating between
meals is also discouraged on the grounds that the body needs sufficient
time to assimilate what is eaten at meal times. The religiously inspired
food practices followed by Seventh Day Adventists, emphasizing cereals,
fruits, vegetables and pulses, has conferred nutritional benefits on them.
As a group they suffer less chronic diet-related disorders such as hyper-
tension and cancer than do the general population.

It is interesting to note in passing, that Dr. John Harvey Kellogg was
for many years responsible for the Sanatorium at Battle Creek, where the
Adventists settled. His attention to the rich and wealthy eventually
brought him into implacable opposition to the White's and he left – but
not before he had established a successful 'health food' trade. One of his
products, cornflakes, was originally seen to be a technologically pure
food, which was therefore pure for the body and the spirit too.

Mormonism

The Mormons, or Latter Day Saints, number about eight million and
claim to be the fastest growing religious organization in the world. About
half of these live in the US and of these, one-third live in Utah. Like the
Seventh Day Adventists, Mormons assert the importance of eating a well-
balanced diet in order to nourish the body as the temple in which the soul
resides. Vegetables and herbs are emphasized while meat should be used
sparingly. Tobacco, alcohol and caffeine are avoided. Mormons recognize
the Sabbath as the day of rest. Organized fasting for those in sound
health occurs once a month; a 24-hour fast lasts from Saturday through to
Sunday evening and money or food saved is contributed to the welfare of
the poor. The fast is a religious discipline and is not a dietary requirement.
Members are also encouraged to fast at times of spiritual need.

Mormons are exhorted to be self-reliant and to prepare for times of
adversity. They are therefore encouraged to keep a home store of 1 year's
supply of food, emphasizing basic items such as grains, legumes, salt,
sugar, powdered milk and cooking oil. Items should be regularly used
and replaced to avoid spoilage and waste (Pike, 1992). Grocery stores in
areas with large Mormon populations tend to sell more bulk packaged
food goods. Generally, intakes of energy, macronutrients, fibre and vitamins A and C among Mormons do not differ from those of the general
population, though milk consumption is high, probably as a consequence

of tea, coffee and alcohol avoidance. Studies in Utah, Alberta and in New Zealand Maoris have shown considerably lower mortality rates among Mormons than in the general population. Lower incidences of heart disease, stroke and cancer may be associated with the tobacco-free, vegetarian lifestyle.

Eastern Orthodoxy

Dietary laws in Eastern Orthodoxy revolve around fasting. There are two major fasts; the Great Lent fast lasts for 40 days preceding Easter, and another 40-day fast occurs in November at Advent. In addition there are two shorter summer fasts and regular fasts on every Wednesday and Friday in the year, except the two before Ascension Day. Fasts do not require total abstinence but rather the foregoing of certain specified foods. All animal products and fish except shellfish are prohibited. Olive oil was historically stored in casks lined with calf's stomach, and was thus viewed as being contaminated through contact with an animal product. The avoidance of such an important food commodity during fast periods is a symbol of true sacrifice and devoutness.

The Great Lent fast commemorates Christ's 40-day fast in the desert. In the 2 or 3 weeks prior to the fast all meat and dairy products in the house are eaten or otherwise disposed of. No animal foods are then eaten until Easter Sunday when the austerity of Lent is ended with the spit-roasting of lambs. On Maundy Thursday lambs are killed and hung in preparation for the resurrection feast. Hard-boiled eggs are dyed red to symbolize Christ's blood. These eggs, symbolizing the tomb of Christ, are considered to be tokens of good luck and are broken open on Easter morning, representing the opening of the tomb. On Good Friday, lentil soup is eaten to symbolize the tears of the Virgin Mary; often it is flavoured with vinegar as a reminder of Christ's ordeal on the cross. The Great Lent fast is broken after a midnight service on Easter Saturday with a lamb-based soup, olives, bread and fruit.

Food symbolism is manifest during these special Easter celebrations, but ritual food is also important in other ceremonies. Special altar bread called Prosphoron – the bread of offering – is prepared by laywomen for use at Sunday Communion. This bread is free from milk, sugar, eggs and shortening, and is stamped with a Prosphoron seal. The centre portion of the loaf represents a lamb and during the Communion becomes transformed into the body of Christ. Other parts of the loaf represent the Virgin Mary and the Angelic Host and Saints. The Prosphoron offering is bought to the altar with two lists of names; one, of living friends and relatives, who are wished good health; and another of the dead, who are wished a peaceful repose.

The New Year ceremony also involves food symbolism. A special bread, Vasilopita is served; it is decorated with blanched almonds which form the first letters of 'Christ', and usually contains a coin which will bring luck to whoever receives the slice containing it. The bread is sliced by the male host and distributed in a ritual order. The first piece is for St Basil; the second is offered to the house as a symbol of prosperity and good fortune; the third is for the male householder and the fourth is given to the oldest female present.

Communion

Though it has been interpreted in various ways and has been given different names (Mass, Eucharist, The Lord's Supper), this celebration has retained an underlying significance as a meal shared by the followers of Jesus. The form of the celebration varies from austere to elaborate but in each case involves the breaking of bread and the sharing of wine. At the Last Supper, Jesus blessed bread and wine and gave it to the disciples saying 'Take this; this is my body' and 'This is my blood, the blood of the covenant.' (Mark 14: 22–24). St. Paul, anxious for converts among Jews, Romans, Greeks and pagans, presented the Last Supper as a sacrifice in which Jesus was the Paschal lamb who was offered up, thereby transferring the symbolism of Passover to the crucifixion.

Doctrinal differences in interpreting the meaning of the Communion meal are found among Christian sects. Whereas Roman Catholics and Eastern Orthodox practitioners believe that the bread and wine actually change to the body and blood of Christ, in a renewed sacrifice by Christ himself, Protestant sects emphasize the remembrance role of the Communion. Some groups, such as the Quakers, have actually forsaken the ritual altogether (cf. Sacraments).

The Baha'i Faith

The Baha'i faith originated with the prophet Baha'u'llah in Iraq in 1863. It now has members in most countries of the world and is one of the fastest-growing religions. It is predicated on a vision of unity and peace for all mankind and enshrines equality and elimination of prejudices as central values.

Food plays a part in the Baha'i religion in three ways; through fasts, through feasts and through dietary injunctions which favour abstention from alcohol, vegetarianism and simplicity. There are also references to other feeding practices contained in letters from Abdu'l-Baha providing guidance to individual believers. For example, mother's milk is explicitly acknowledged to be the preferred way of feeding infants. There are some obvious parallels with Islamic practices, not surprisingly, given the geographical origin of the faith. Fasting is viewed as a spiritual undertaking and is symbolic of abstinence from selfish and carnal desires. It is deemed to have both physical and spiritual benefits.

A 19-day fasting period occurs in March, during which there must be complete abstention from food and drink between sunrise and sunset. This echoes the Moslem fast of Ramadhan and, also as in Islam, exemptions are granted for travellers, the sick, pregnant and nursing women. Those engaged in heavy work may also be excused. Children under the age of 15 years and elderly persons over 70 years of age are not required to fast. Those exempted may, if they so choose, participate in the fast. Obeying the fast is a matter for individual conscience and is not enforced; if food is eaten 'unconsciously' during the fast it is deemed to be an accident rather than a breaking of the fast. Unlike in Islam, there is no making up of fast days missed as the fast can only be kept during the designated time.

'Feast', in the Baha'i faith, has a particular meaning which incorporates spiritual, business and social elements. Local Spiritual Assemblies hold Nineteen-Day Feasts (so-called because they are held on the first day of each of the 19-day-long Baha'i months), at which Baha'is gather to consult and discuss and to offer suggestions to the Local Spiritual Assembly. At a feast, which is entered into with right thinking, the heavenly food of knowledge, understanding, love and kindness is present, providing members with a sense of spiritual restoration. Thus administrative and spiritual purposes are blended. Non-Baha'is may attend feasts (though they should not be specifically invited to do so), but in such cases the consultative part of the proceedings is omitted. Where Local Spiritual Assemblies do not exist groups of Baha'is may gather for a feast which omits the formal administrative element described above.

Feasts are held either in formal worship centres or in homes of the Assembly members. In the latter case, the host provides the food and must personally serve the other members. As the numbers of people involved may be large, the obligation to provide food for all may create a considerable financial burden for hosts. However, the hosting role rotates among members and is therefore relatively infrequent for any one. Also, the food provided may be very simple – for example, biscuits and water – and so costs can be minimized. The significance of providing food at the gathering appears to be related to the Baha'i injunction to serve one's fellows rather than to the social solidarity of sharing food. The absence of guidelines or restrictions on what may be served indicates that it is the act of serving which is symbolic, not the food itself.

There are a number of guidelines relating to diet, some of which come direct from the writings of Baha'u'llah and others which originate with Abdu'l-Baha. As in many cultural traditions, diet is seen to be integral to well-being and the differentiation between diet and medicine is blurred. Thus Baha'is are exhorted to treat disease through diet whenever possible though drugs are not to be avoided if they are necessary. Principles of allopathic medicine are adduced to promote the healing of illness by food. Thus, Baha'u'llah taught that disease is caused by an imbalance of bodily components and the aim of the physician is to discover what the imbalance is and to prescribe the correct foods to restore the equilibrium. Calling on the example of animals in the wild, it is further suggested that the human body knows what foods it needs to restore imbalances, but that our as yet imperfect medical science has not grasped the fact. Nevertheless, Baha'is are encouraged to consult and subscribe to the ministrations of competent physicians.

The virtue of moderation is upheld by preferring that meals consist of only one course, which should if possible be of good quality. Simplicity in eating is also a way of freeing people from their appetites and of improving health through diminishing chronic disease. This parallels the idea of spiritual simplicity which is thought to improve the moral character and conduct of people. Vegetarianism is held to be a compassionate practice and one which is in line with God's will and though meat is not prohibited it is seen to be unnecessary. Whereas God equipped predatory animals with talons and claws to obtain meat, and grazing animals with teeth suitable to eating vegetables:

> But now coming to man, we see he hath neither hooked teeth nor sharp nails or claws, nor teeth like iron sickles. From this it becometh evident and manifest that the food of man is cereals and fruit. Some of the teeth of man are like millstones to grind the grain, and some are sharp to cut the fruit. Therefore, he is not in need of meat, nor is he obliged to eat it. Even without meat he would live with the utmost vigour and energy.
>
> *Abdu'l-Baha, quoted in Hornby (1988)*

In a similar way, the killing of animals is not prohibited but is not favoured. Abdu'l-Baha's prediction that the time would come when meat would no longer be eaten has interesting resonances with Norbert Elias' notion of the curve of civilization (cf. techniques of eating). In a social context, Baha'is should follow the guiding principles of moderation and courtesy in deciding whether to refuse food offered to them or to request special food.

Islam

The meaning of Islam is 'submission', and for millions of devout Moslems around the world it is a way of life: a religion which intimately affects law, morality and social relations. Islam is one of the youngest of the major religions and the second largest in the world, with adherents among nearly all cultures. There are a multitude of different sects, exhibiting varying degrees of orthodoxy.

Moslems believe that the founder of their religion, Mohammed, was the last of God's prophets; they accept the divinity of the teachings of earlier prophets but believe that the Bible was superseded by the Qur'an, a Holy Book given to Mohammed by Allah. Mohammed would have been familiar with Israelite history and customs, and this, together with the geographical proximity of the two religious worlds and the presence in the deserts of Arabia of heretic Christians driven out of Rome, has resulted in certain similarities between Jewish and Islamic practices.

All foods are permitted (**halal**) with a few exceptions that are specifically prohibited (**haram**). A chapter of the Qur'an known as the Surah contains dietary regulations. In addition, the authenticated sayings and actions of the prophet Mohammed are recorded in the Hadith wherein are found hundreds of reports of what Mohammed ate, gave to others or said about food on various occasions. Flesh of animals that are cloven hoofed and those that chew the cud is lawful. Pigs, blood, carrion and foods offered to other idols are forbidden, though one who eats these foods under constraint does not sin. Carnivorous animals and birds which seize their prey with talons are forbidden, as is the flesh of the domestic ass. Alcohol is prohibited. Fish must be alive when taken from the sea or river, and only fish which have fins and scales are allowed thus excluding shellfish and eels. Land animals without ears, such as frogs and snakes are prohibited. Food is a gift from God and should not be wasted. To be acceptable to a Moslem an animal must be bled to death while the words 'Bismi 'llahi. Allah Akbar' (I begin with God's name. God is great) are spoken. Such meat is stamped with a Halal seal. In the US, food products which conform to Islamic law may be identified with a Crescent M symbol.

The religious practices of Moslems are guided by the Five Pillars of Islam. These are faith, prayer, alms giving, fasting and pilgrimage to Mecca. Prayers are said regularly throughout the day. If no mosque is nearby, a devout Moslem will kneel on his personal prayer-rug, facing Mecca, and pray. Moslems are expected to give a proportion of their wealth, in money or livestock, as **Zakat**. Originally intended to support the poor, Zakat is often used to support mosques and schools, especially in non-Moslem countries. The pilgrimage to Mecca is the often once-in-a-lifetime trip made by devout Moslems from all over the world. The great Mosque there holds over 35 000 people, and a 100-square mile area around Mecca is closed to all who are not Moslems. Fasting, or **sawm**, is an important duty. It is a way of expressing piety, self-restraint and freedom from worldly desire, and is a means of reaping spiritual rewards. Except for a few holy festival days Moslems may voluntarily fast whenever they wish. Mohammed said, 'Every good act that a man does shall receive from ten to seven hundred rewards, but the rewards of fasting are beyond bounds for fasting is for God alone and He will give its rewards'. Strict adherents fast on Monday and Thursday of every week and on the 13th, 14th and 15th of each month. Shi'i Moslems fast to commemorate the martyrdom of Ali, son-in-law of the Prophet, and his two sons.

Ramadhan, falling in the ninth lunar month, is the major fast of the Moslem year. The word is derived from **ramz**, meaning to burn, and may derive either from the fact that the fast was first observed in the hot season, or because it was believed that fasting would burn away sins. The Ramadhan fast involves abstinence from food and water between sunrise and sunset for the whole month, and is prescribed for all who have reached the Age of Responsibility, (12 years for girls; 15 years for boys). The desire to participate in the fast is encouraged in children from as young as 6 to 8 years of age. Special dishes are prepared to celebrate **roza khushai**, the day of a child's first fast. Traditionally, eating and drinking is permitted during the night until dawn when a white thread can be distinguished from a black one, though a standard time is now often employed. The day's fast should be broken as soon after sunset as possible by a snack known as **iftari**. An evening meal follows and this often takes place at a mosque or at house parties, for it is highly commendable to provide food to others, especially the poor. Lebanese Moslems often eat Fattoush, a mixed salad, to break the day of fasting. A predawn meal known as **sehri** should be eaten as late as is possible prior to sunrise.

The Ramadhan fast is one of the most strictly observed of Islamic practices. Deliberate infractions necessitate **qada**, or restitution, in which missed days are made up as soon as possible, and also **kaffarah**, or atonement, which involves prolonged additional fasting, extensive feeding of the poor or the freeing of a Moslem slave. Different sects have different laws and customs regarding qada and kaffarah. Certain groups are exempted partially or totally from the Ramadhan fast. Anyone who is sick, on a journey, or engaged in hard labour may break the fast, but must make up the days later. This applies also to women who are menstruating or are in childbirth. Pregnant or nursing women and elderly persons in poor health may defer fasting until later in the year or may 'substitute fast' by feeding the poor. Younger children are expected to undertake short fasts in preparation for when they reach the Age of Responsibility. The end of Ramadhan is signalled by the sighting of the new moon, and is celebrated with prayers and with feasting in a festival called Id-ul-Fitr. There is large scale communal prayer, much visiting of friends and relatives and to graves of ancestors, and giving of charity and small money gifts to young people in family.

Id is associated with the serving of sweet foods and is commonly known as 'sweet Id'. Sawaiyan is a fine vermicelli, boiled and served with milk and sugar. It epitomizes sweet dishes, food sharing, equality and hospitality for guests, and is the symbol of the festival (Murphy, 1986). On Id it is said that everyone is God's guest; therefore to fast on Id is haram.

Id-ul-Azha or bakra Id is celebrated two and a half months later when the annual pilgrimage to Mecca is under way. In contrast to sweet Id, bakra Id features a blood sacrifice, called **qurbani**, the purpose of which is commemoration of Abraham's willingness to sacrifice his son at God's command. The sacrifice fulfils a religious obligation and gives the person in whose name it is made, **sawab**, or meritorious reward from God. Liver, lungs and heart are the first edible parts removed from the animal and are used to prepare kaleji which can be used to break the fast which orthodox Moslems keep on this day prior to the sacrifice. Islamic prescriptions require that the sacrificial meat be divided into three equal portions; one for the family, one for friends, relatives and neighbours, and one for charity (Murphy, 1986).

Judaism

The first five books of the Old Testament, known collectively as the Torah, contain what are probably the most detailed dietary directions of any major religion. These biblical injunctions have been interpreted, elaborated and added to by rabbis over the past 2000 years. The term, **kashruth**, meaning acceptable, is used to describe anything permitted by Jewish dietary laws. Such laws are concerned with prohibition of whole or parts of animals, methods of slaughter, and with preparation techniques – including mixing of certain food products. Foods which are unclean or not properly prepared are termed **trayf**.

Kashruth

Only animals having cloven hooves and that chew the cud are permitted. Thus cows, sheep, oxen and goats may be eaten whereas pigs, hares and camels may not be. Permitted fish must have fins and scales, which excludes shellfish. Other forbidden foods include teeming winged insects, except locusts, certain birds of prey and bats. To avoid confusion and to obviate the need to make difficult discriminations between animals, the prohibition was later extended by the rabbis to include all insects and birds of prey. Neither blood nor internal organ fat of otherwise permitted animals may be eaten. The sciatic nerve may not be eaten and, as its removal is difficult, often only the forequarters of an animal is used. The rest of the meat may be sold to non-Jews. Rabbinic additions to the Biblical laws decreed that milk from non-kosher animals is forbidden as it has the same qualities as the animal from which it comes.

Animals dying of natural causes or of disease are not permitted for consumption. Meat must be obtained from animals which have been ritually slaughtered under the supervision of a rabbi. A trained butcher, or **shochet**, slashes the animal's throat with a single cut so as to allow the blood to drain completely from the body. The animal is examined for internal irregularities which might render it unfit for consumption and, if acceptable, is given a seal of approval. Following slaughter, soaking, draining and salting of the meat ensures that all traces of blood are removed. Once a domestic task, this is now usually done commercially and the shochet has become the modern equivalent of the priest who controlled animal sacrifices in the Temple of Jerusalem. Historically, Jewish migration was dependent on the availability of kosher meat and thus of access to the services of a shochet. Berman (1982) provides a detailed list of the characteristics required in a shochet as well as the duties the position entails.

A prohibition against mixing meat and dairy products is based on the biblical injunction 'You shall not boil a kid in its mother's milk.' (Exodus 23:19). After eating milk, hand washing and mouth rinsing is all that is necessary before eating meat; however, depending on local custom, from 1 to 6 hours must elapse after eating meat and before eating milk. Margarine and milk and cream substitutes have made this particular law easier to follow: nevertheless many observant Jews view the use of such substitutes as being spiritually wrong.

Processed foods may contain ingredients which are not acceptable under the kosher laws and kosher foods have become big business. It is estimated that more than 21 000 kosher-supervised products are now available, that 30% of products found in a typical US supermarket are labelled kosher, and that traditional kosher consumers constitute only about a quarter of the kosher market. Moslems, Seventh Day Adventists, vegetarians and the lactose-intolerant may also use kosher markings to guide their dietary choices (Regenstein and Regenstein, 1992). There are several ways to determine whether a product is kosher. The label may state that the product is kosher, or a letter K, U, MKU or COR may appear. There may be a kosher supervisory agency's symbol on the product or the seller may display such a symbol identifying that all products sold in the store meet the kosher standards of the supervisory agency. Common infringements of kosher standards include; the presence in a store of forbidden foods such as pork or shellfish; the passing off of cheaper non-kosher meat and cheese as kosher; the commingling of sealed packages of kosher and non-kosher meats on store shelves; changes in production practices which render a kosher product non-kosher; use of a kosher symbol on a non-kosher product; handling procedures such as cutting kosher meat on a non-kosher slicer. Fruits and vegetables might be coated with animal-based materials or be contaminated by insects. Regenstein and Regenstein discuss these issues in detail, identifying the key problem as lack of written standards for kosher products.

Berman (1982), who is critical of the kosher labelling enterprise, points out that the kosher symbol is placed on foods which don't need it, just to provide a competitive edge in the supermarket. He draws parallels between the big-business orientation of modern kashruth practices and the ancient excesses of Temple sacrifice, and declares that because of the often cruel methods of animal rearing employed, approved meats are kosher in name only.

Observance of the laws of Kashruth varies both between and within the various Jewish sects. While Reform Jews have abandoned many of the dietary restrictions as being anachronistic, ultra-orthodox Hasidic Jews have maintained and even strengthened those laws, thus setting themselves apart within the faith as well as from wider society. Conservative Jews strike a compromise, forsaking some of the stricter orthodox ways but continuing to eat kosher foods. Transgressions of dietary laws are sanctioned and encouraged if health is at risk.

Feasts, fasts and holidays

All Jewish festivals are religious in nature and all have historical significance, many being reminders of past persecution. In this way they provide a sense of continuity with the past as well as of ethnic solidarity with co-religionists around the world. Symbolism is rife in festive food practices. There are many fasts in the Jewish calendar, some of scriptural or rabbinical origin and others which mark private events such as family deaths. Fasting is a way of showing repentance, of teaching self-discipline, or of preparing to seek divine guidance. Generally fasts are observed by boys over the age of 13 years and 1 day, and by girls over the age of 12 years and 1 day.

The Sabbath being a day of rest, all food preparation is carried out on Friday. Challah is a traditional Sabbath bread and, in a modern adaptation of an historical practice, two loaves are used to symbolize the double portion of manna provided by God to the Israelites on Fridays during their 40 years in the wilderness. Rosh Hashannah, the Day of Judgement, is the Jewish New Year festival. Sweet foods such as apple slices dipped in honey are eaten to symbolize faith in God's mercy and the prospect of a good year. Ten days later comes Yom Kippur, the Day of Atonement, on which a complete fast lasting dusk to dusk is undertaken. A full meal should be eaten on the eve of Yom Kippur so that the pain of fasting will be all the more acute. At this meal, meat-filled dumplings known as kreplach are served, which represent stern judgement wrapped in mercy.

In preparation for the major festival of Passover all leavened products must be removed from the house, reflecting the fact that Jews did not have time to let bread dough rise when they were driven from their homes into exile. Pieces of bread may be deliberately hidden around the house, to be discovered and removed. Unleavened bread called **matzah** is prepared or bought commercially. On the eve of Passover it is customary for the oldest child to fast in symbolic remembrance of the historic sparing of the first-born. On the first and second night a special family meal, the seder, is eaten, which is an elaborate testimony to the symbolic power of food. Seder means order, and the meal indeed has a very definite structure which gives it its ritual character. A food event thus becomes an important way of transmitting culturally valued knowledge from generation to generation.

The seder

During the seder meal a collection of stories and prayers known as the Haggadah is read. Foods on the seder dish are eaten at specific points during this reading. Three matzah, each covered with a cloth, represent the three estates of Israel and also recall the three measures of meal which Sarah, wife of Abraham, prepared for the three angels who visited on the night of Passover. At the beginning of the meal the middle matzah is broken to symbolize the parting of the Red Sea. Half is eaten and half, the afiquoman, is set aside to be eaten just before Grace so that the taste of freedom will linger in the mouth. Maror, or bitter herbs (usually a piece of horseradish) represent the bitterness of slavery in Egypt; karpas – greens such as celery, parsley or watercress – recall the poor diet there endured. Haroseth, prepared differently by Jewish communities around the world, is a mixture of chopped fruit and nuts mixed with cinnamon and wine or grape juice, which represents the clay or mortar used by the slaves to make bricks, but which also recalls the sweetness of redemption. It is shaped into small balls or spread on matzahs. A dish of salt water into which the parsley is dipped symbolizes the tears of the oppressed. A roast shank bone recalls the sacrifice of the Paschal lamb at the Temple of Jerusalem, while a roast egg stands for a second animal sacrifice. Four cups of wine are drunk during the meal, recalling the four promises of redemption given in Exodus, and a fifth cup is filled for the prophet Elijah who is said to visit every Jewish home on this night. The afiquoman may be hidden for the children to find, a small prize being given to the winner.

Hinduism

Originating in India over four millennia ago, Hinduism is usually considered to be the oldest living religion. The word is a corruption of **Sindhu** and means 'the people and culture of the Indus river region' – indicating its geographic origin. The Aryan invasion of North West India in about 2150 BCE gave Hinduism its modern cultural and mythic form, written down as a series of hymns or scriptures known as the Vedas. Over the centuries India, and Hinduism, was influenced by a wide range of other cultures and religious movements. 'Beginning with the Indo–Aryan hybridization, India has been influenced by Persians, Zoroastrians, Buddhists, Jains, Greeks, Macedonians, Arabs, Mongols, Sikhs, Portuguese, French, Dutch, Mughals, and the British.' (Kilara and Iya, 1992).

It is thus not surprising that Hinduism synthesizes many diverse beliefs, and that Hindus worship a multitude of deities; though all of them are part of the one supreme Universal Spirit, Brahman, who pervades and upholds the structure of the universe.

Brahman originally created the Universe as the God, Brahma; as Vishnu he sustained the Universe, then as Shiva he destroyed it. The Universe is thus cyclical. The present Universe was created by Brahma and will in time be destroyed again by Shiva. On an individual level too, the Hindu views life as a process of renewal, firmly believing that past and future reincarnations reflect on one's spiritual progress.

Pervading Hindu life is the social structure known as the caste system. Like class, caste is something one is born into, but unlike class one has no opportunity to move across caste boundaries in one's present lifetime. Caste is determined by actions in previous lives and is thus accepted with a surprising degree of fatalism and docility. Social injustice, poverty and discrimination can thus be reconciled, even by those who suffer most. The caste system arose from the four Vedic estates or varnas; according to a creation myth, Purusa, who was an original Divine whose body filled the universe, was sacrificed by the Gods. Parts of his body formed the various elements of Creation. The highest caste, the Brahmin, sprang from Purusa's mouth. Originally, Brahmin were priests and teachers and were not permitted to take up any other type of work. They were supported in food and money by members of other castes, who attracted merit to themselves by the act of giving. Modern-day Brahmins often hold powerful professional and business positions. From Purusa's arms came the Ksatriyas, the rulers and the warriors. They were expected to take the role of protecting the community, and particularly the Brahmins, with their lives if necessary. They were allowed to kill animals and were meat eaters. The Vaisyas, farmers and traders, were formed from Purusa's thighs; their duty was to support the community economically. The Sudras came from the God's feet; they were the menial labourers whose duty was to serve the other three castes. There was some degree of social mobility and social intercourse between the divisions. The system of Varna was codified in the Law of Manu during the second century CE. It coincided with a hardening of social divisions in society, and the rights and duties of the four estates became markedly differentiated. Numerous castes developed within the varna framework – including the Untouchables, who were often denied even menial work, and who were banned from the villages and towns. Most castes are subdivided and are closed social groups who practise endogamy, thus reinforcing the caste divisions. Although they maintain a social independence, because of a strict demarcation of jobs the various castes are in fact extremely interdependent and are indispensable to each other. This system resembles to a degree, the feudal relationships extant in Medieval Europe. Although Mahatma Gandhi struggled to end the concept of untouchability and although it was officially declared illegal in 1949, the concept of impenetrable social barriers remains strong. Only by leading a high moral existence in one life can one be reborn at a higher level in the next; one's future is the direct consequence of one's current actions.

Whereas vegetarianism and the specific prohibition on eating cows are two of the dietary hallmarks of modern Hinduism, this was not always the case. Early Hindu writings reveal that beef eating was practised and it can therefore be deduced that the prohibition only arose later, possibly as a response to the challenge of Buddhism. It was perhaps subsequently strengthened by the need for Hindus to distinguish themselves from their new Moslem neighbours. Certainly by the time of the Rigveda, around 1000 CE, the prohibition was firmly ensconced.

Dietary laws were recorded in the Code of Manu in the second century BCE (Table 6.3). Over 200 foods and food-related activities are forbidden as being unwholesome. This includes specific prohibited foods, rules on who may have access to or receive food from whom, rituals that define food purity, and behaviours which compromise purity. Meat eating is not prohibited but is discouraged; for meat cannot be obtained without injuring a sentient being, which action is an impediment to attaining heavenly bliss. The Code of Manu allows for dietary restrictions to be relaxed if conditions are such that survival is threatened. Echoes of this are seen in modern India, where observance of prohibitions is strictest in the upper Brahmin caste while beef eating is tolerated among lower castes, for whom it may be an important source of supplementary protein.

Table 6.3 Dietary regulations outlined in the Hindu Code of Manu

---

- Wound not others, do not injury by thought or deed, utter no word to pain thy fellow creatures

- One should cease from eating all flesh. There is no fault in eating flesh, nor in drinking intoxicating liquor, nor in copulation, for that is the occupation of beings, but cessation from them produces great fruit

- Meat can never be obtained without injury to living creatures, and injury to sentient beings is detrimental to the attainment of heavenly bliss

- There is no greater sinner than that man who, though not worshipping the Gods or the manes, seeks to increase the bulk of his own flesh by the flesh of other beings

---

The caste system is an excellent example of the way in which social structures influence food practices. Concepts of purity and pollution determine who may eat what with whom and who may accept what food from whom. Eating with or accepting food from members of a lower class is polluting. In the hot–cold classification system used in traditional healing, raw foods are considered to be hot and are therefore purer than cooked foods, which are cold. Brahmins who accept food cooked by a lower caste person lose ritual purity and thus caste status; however, they may accept raw materials for a meal and also ghee and milk, for these are products of the sacred cow and cannot be polluted by touch. Wealthy families may keep two kitchens, one for Brahmins and one for non-Brahmins, with separate cooking and eating utensils and, sometimes, even separate cooks. In Northern India, foods are categorized as being pukka or kacca (kutcha). Kacca foods are cooked without fat (rice, chapatties) and are most vulnerable to impurity. Pukka foods are deep fried in ghee and are therefore insulated against impurities and pollution. Kacca food is used as ordinary family fare and as payment for servants and artisans (Kilara and Iya, 1992).

Hospitality, and moderation in eating are cardinal principles for Hindus. Devout Hindus are vegetarian, though the interpretation of this varies somewhat by caste and region. Meat, fish and often eggs are avoided, the latter especially by women, though Brahmins in Northern India will often eat meat. For example, the Gadulia Lohar, a major nomadic community, although claiming a Ksatriya caste status do not pay much attention to concepts of purity and pollution unless they are Bhagats, or devotees. Generally they eat meat and drink alcohol (Misra, 1986). Fish avoidance was probably introduced by fish-avoiding Aryans who invaded northern India around 1500 BCE (Simoons, 1974). The taboo is seen among peoples living alongside these ancient migration routes, but not in other areas. Where fish is eaten, white fish is preferred for it is least like meat.

Feasts, fasts and festivals

There are literally thousands of festival days celebrated by Hindus in different parts of India. Some are national, some regional and some purely local. On festival days there may be great processions and people visit the shrine of the feted deity where they pray and make offerings. Food which has been offered to a god is thereby blessed, and is distributed to an eager crowd. Ghee (clarified butter), as a product of the cow, is sacred and is an important component of many rituals. For example, during marriage ceremonies a ritual flame is kept burning with ghee. **Shaadh** (desire) is a celebration to honour a woman who is going to give birth to her first child. The mother-in-law invites married female friends and relatives to a meal to mark the fifth, seventh and ninth months of the pregnancy, at which time she serves five, seven and nine different dishes respectively. The pregnant woman may eat whatever she desires. The tradition is widespread even in the poorest villages. It is important to satisfy the mother-to-be's desires so that if she should die in childbirth her soul will rest in peace. The modern Indian festivals of Dussatra and Divali illustrate the agricultural origins of many contemporary celebrations. Dussatra marks the end of the rainy season when agricultural labour must begin anew, as well as commemorating the legendary hero, Rama. It includes a ritual quest for alms by people carrying small fresh stalks of barley plants. Divali, known as the festival of lights, is a New-Year festival celebrating the sowing of winter crops. Lamps are lit and gifts are exchanged.

Abstention from eating food is a much praised virtue. Some Hindus may fast 2 or 3 days a week during which time they may eat only pure foods such as milk, fruit, nuts, starchy roots and vegetables. Fasts are associated with calendric, caste, family and personal events as well as with religious celebrations.

Jainism

Jainism is an ascetic religion whose adherents advocate **ahimsa**, or non-injury, both as an ethical and philosophical goal; not only killing, but any form of aggression is shunned. The Jaina monastic community has a number of characteristic practices which evince an extreme regard for life. Monks carry a small brush with which they carefully sweep the floor before sitting or lying so as to avoid crushing any insects. A mask may be worn to prevent inadvertent inhalation of small creatures, and water is strained for the same reason. Ascetics have few or no possessions and must beg for food. Some choose in old age to die through ritual fasting.

Most Jainas are not ascetics, though some strive to imitate monastic ideals by pursuing a progressive path of renunciation, leading to rebirth as an ascetic. The non-monastic Jaina community practises vegetarianism and opposes the killing of animals. Because of this, agricultural and military occupations are not suitable to Jainas, who historically have chosen instead to enter the professions or to take up business interests. As a result they became a wealthy group who were able to financially support the cultural institutions necessary to teach and preserve their traditions.

Sikhism

Sikh means disciple, a follower of the ten gurus. Sikhism was founded in the 15th century CE by the guru Nanak who proclaimed 'There is no Hindu; there is no Moslem'. Nanak rejected the social distinctions of the Hindu caste system and idol worship. Those who sought him out as a teacher had first to eat in a communal kitchen, or **dhamsala**, where Moslems and Hindus of all castes sat side-by-side to eat. By requiring his disciples to share food Nanak had found a practical way to create the unity he espoused. Following Nanak came nine more gurus the last of whom, Gobind Singh, established the distinctive male Sikh practice of wearing a turban and beard and carrying a ceremonial dagger. In addition he forbade tobacco and alcohol use to converts, as well as meat from animals which had been bled to death. All Sikhs take the name Singh, which means lion.

Sikhs retain the Hindu reverence for cows, and thus do not eat beef. Other meat may be eaten though some Sikhs are vegetarians. Permitted animals must be killed with a single blow known as **jhatka**, literally a sudden shake or jerk. Generally, Sikhs are not rigid about adherence to dietary laws, and readily adapt to the food customs of other cultures.

Buddhism

Buddhism developed as an offshoot from, and in turn influenced, Hinduism. Founded in the sixth century BCE by Siddartha Gautama, Buddhism became the state religion of India in 250 BCE, though it is now a minority religion there. Buddhism has developed in different ways in many parts of the world and is predominant in Japan, Taiwan, Cambodia, Laos, Thailand, Sri Lanka and Burma. There are 100 million Buddhists in China and about half a million in North America.

Buddha taught the Four Noble Truths. Existence is suffering; this suffering is due to selfish desires; the cure of suffering is to destroy these selfish desires; this cure can be effected by following the eight-fold path of right action, right speech, right livelihood, right effort, right mindfulness, right concentration, right views, right intentions. Eliminating individual desires by following the eight-way path of righteousness is the way for Buddhists to attain Nirvana. This may take several reincarnations during which progress is made through Right Action. Such Right Action includes refraining from eating meat or from harming any living creatures, though the prohibition is observed strictly only by monks and the devout laity. No solid food may be eaten in the afternoon. 'Five pungent foods', garlic, scallion, leek, chives and onion are to be avoided as they create strong emotions which interfere with the purification of the mind. Lay Buddhists may occasionally eat meat, or may raise meat for sale to non-Buddhists. Animals found dead may be eaten, as may fish (which are not 'killed' but merely removed from the water). In contrast to dietary prohibitions of other religions, emphasis is placed on wrongful killing rather than wrongful eating. The twin concepts of **karma**, or moral conduct and **karuna**, or compassion underlie Buddhist vegetarian practices. To eat the flesh of an animal is to destroy the seeds of compassion, or karuna; conversely, avoiding meat will lead to the development of a compassionate heart. The karmic concept that good is rewarded by good and evil with evil leads to the belief that a life destroyed must be payed for with life, and thus the path to Nirvana is delayed.

As in Jainism, the monks personify the ideal. Food is obtained through begging and it is meritorious for the laity to voluntarily provide food to the monks, thereby assisting in their own spiritual progress. As the monastic population in Buddhist countries has declined, so too has the burden on villagers who support them. For example, with the Chinese-inspired secularization of Tibet, Buddhist monks have become more involved in agricultural work to support themselves. Crop production takes precedence over animal rearing because of the emphasis on the non-taking of life. Animals may occasionally be eaten by lay Buddhists, or raised and sold to Chinese merchants.

Shinto

Shinto is the traditional religion of Japan which has persisted from ancient times; many modern Japanese simultaneously practise both Shinto and Buddhism. Shinto is a polytheistic religion dedicated to the way of **kami** and is in essence a worship of nature. Kamis are supernatural beings, many of whom are nature gods. Pre-eminent is the sun goddess, but next in importance is Uke-mochi, the food goddess. Inasi, the rice god, is a variant of Uke-mochi. There are extensive communal and private shrines to Inasi, who grants his worshippers agricultural prosperity.

Numerous festivals have evolved, the two most important of which are Toshigobi, the Spring Prayer for Harvests (and latterly, success in industrial enterprise), and Tsukinami, the Fall festival of Thanksgiving for the protection of the gods. Traditionally at these festivals rice, salt, sake, fruit and vegetables would be provided for the kami to share. Such offerings were ways of paying respects and receiving the kami's blessings. The custom of offering cooked food to share with the kami is still observed in the Shinto shrines of the Imperial household. Elsewhere, only uncooked food is offered, not to share, but simply as supplication or thanksgiving.

North American religions

Diverse cultural traditions are found among the aboriginal peoples of North America reflecting differing beliefs, myths and ceremonies. Two examples will be used to illustrate religious food practices in a hunting–fishing region and an agricultural region. North-West Coast Indian culture offers a rich array of food-related rituals. Belief in reincarnation and the transmigration of souls into animals demands that a proper universal balance be maintained by ensuring that not only humans, but also animals and spirits, receive the food and souls they require. First Salmon rites were important occasions at which propitiatory rituals were held in order to guarantee continued food security. A salmon chief would greet the first salmon, honouring it with speeches and ensuring that after death it was prepared with due respect. As a consequence, the freed soul of the salmon would return to inform other salmon of the proper treatment it received, and thus ensure continued future supplies of food. Similarly, people of the Gitksan tribe would throw beaver bones back into the river so that the beaver would re-inhabit it. For the Gitksan, the arrival of the first Spring salmon triggered a solemn ceremony of gratitude. The first fish were carried ceremoniously to the village and each fish was laid out on a separate clean woven cedar mat. Eagle down was sprinkled on the fish and another clean mat was placed on top. No one in the village spoke during the entire night but the next morning there was an expression of thanks. The fish were then cooked whole and cut into portions so that every man, child and eligible woman received a piece. Songs and dances to give thanks probably accompanied this distribution (People of 'Ksan 1980).

For Indians of the South-West, the introduction of maize in the third millennium BCE had immense consequences. Social organization and religious rites changed to meet the needs of an agricultural way of life. The newly important agricultural spirits had to be placated and sacrifices, which had never been an important part of Indian culture, were needed to ensure crop fertility. Among the Hopi Indians maize is a dominant symbol of life. All parts of the maize – ears, seeds, tassels, milk and pollen – figure in various rituals. A newborn child is presented with two ears of white maize, its 'mothers'; ears of blue maize accompany the dead on their journey beyond life. Cornmeal is a purifying substance which accompanies all private and public prayers. It is sprinkled on kachina dancers to form spiritual paths for the dead, and is offered to the sun and to still-growing maize plants to encourage their successful maturation.

African religions

Indigenous African religions developed prior to the advent of Christianity and Islam and, where they persist, exhibit great diversity from region to region. African traditional religions centre on ancestor worship; one of the most important rituals is that of animal sacrifice. Sacrifice is associated with the agricultural calendar, with medical curative needs and with divination rituals. Animals with specific characteristics, of colour or size for example, are more or less suitable for specific deities, and are offered in return for blessings or perhaps to effect cures or avert death in one who is ill (when the illness may be transferred to the sacrificial animal.) The act of sacrifice performs a dual function of establishing a bond between humans and their deities, and of reinforcing the social solidarity of the human group.

SUMMARY

Whatever their origins, religious dietary requirements can serve a number of purposes. Food mediates communication with God or the supreme being. On a spiritual level adherence to food rules demonstrates faith and rejection of worldliness; on an earthly level, discreet food habits create a sense of identity or belongingness with co-religionists and express separateness from others. Religious injunctions may arise from or serve to reinforce ecologically desirable practices. In some ancient religions food customs and regulations have changed over time as the religion has been influenced by and made accommodations to new social and spiritual movements.

Normative religious food practices are not observed uniformly by adherents of the faith. Variations occur depending on age, sex, social status, geographical region, degree of acculturation and many other factors. Today there seems to be a general decline in the power of traditional religious beliefs. Whereas in some countries taboos remain strong, proscriptions against the eating of particular foods are being generally weakened and in many areas of the world only the priesthood and the devout laity fully observe them.

FURTHER READING

Khare, R.S. and Rao, M.S.A. (eds) (1986) *Food, Society, and Culture*, Carolina Academic Press, North Carolina. The essay by Murphy provides a case study of Moslem food habits in a Hindu-dominated cultural milieu. Toomey, writing in the same collection, explores the differing nature of caste and food usage among two Hindu sects.

Kilara and Iya (1992) provide details of historical and contemporary food habits among Hindus, while Simoons (1961) gives a fascinating account of the origins and the spread of pork avoidance in the Old World, illustrating the effect of successive waves of conquerors on the beliefs and practices of peoples in different areas.

For studies of disease incidence among Mormons, see Enstrom, J.E. (1989) Health practices and mortality among active Californian Mormons, *J. Natl. Cancer Inst.*, **81**: 1807–14; and Jarvis, G.K. (1977) Mormon mortality rates in Canada, *Social Biol.*, **24**: 294–302.

For recent studies of the health of Seventh Day Adventists see Fønnebø, V. (1994) The healthy Seventh-day Adventist lifestyle: what is the Norwegian experience?, *Am. J. Clin. Nutr.*, **59**(suppl): S1124–9; and Mills, P.K., Beeson, W.L., Phillips, R.L. and Fraser, G.E. (1994) Cancer Incidence among California Seventh-day Adventists, 1976–1982, *Am. J. Clin. Nutr.*, **59**(suppl): S1136–42.

DISCUSSION QUESTIONS

1. For a selected religion describe the major functions of its food ideology and practices.
2. Compare the nature and functions of fasting in different religious traditions.
3. Discuss the impact of religion on nutritional status.

4. Provide examples of religious food practices which exacerbate and which minimize social differences between co-religionists.
5. To what extent do you think religious food practices influence eating habits in contemporary society? What are your reasons for thinking this and how might you go about finding out if your views are accurate?
6. Discuss the notion that food can be nutritious but not satisfying.

CHAPTER 7

Morals, ethics, cultism and quackery

Without necessarily claiming any religious motivation it is possible to invoke reasons of morality to support particular eating habits. A good example of this is the whole business of non-meat-eating. Although non-meat-eating is a characteristic of several religions it is a practice also enthusiastically embraced by many who would not consider themselves religious in the nominal sense of the word. Moral attitudes also influence other aspects of food behaviour such as types of food eaten and amount of money spent on food, and are expressed in the contrasting philosophies of 'eating to live' and 'living to eat'.

Food cultism is a term used, somewhat pejoratively, to describe patterns of eating which are either unusual or based on pseudo-scientific reasoning. Cultism may be centred around the supposed efficacy of one particular dietary substance or may involve quite complex patterns of food behaviour. A cult often assumes a pseudo-religious mantle among its followers, and indeed has some common ground with orthodox religions in that faith is usually a strong characteristic of its adherents. While many food cultists have a genuine commitment to the pursuit of health and well-being, others are out-and-out quacks, using pseudo-scientific ideas to peddle pet theories and to thereby turn a quick profit through exploitation of human credulity.

MORALS AND ETHICS

Is it wrong to eat certain foods, even if they are culturally acceptable and are not restricted by religious taboos? Some people certainly think so, and the case of non-meat-eating is discussed at length below. Other foods or food products may be occasionally singled out by individuals or groups as being morally unacceptable because of the way in which they are produced or marketed. Such was the case with South African food products which were heavily boycotted by anti-apartheid supporters in the 1960s and 1970s. The foods themselves were not of course the source of moral contention, but rather they were chosen as symbols of what was viewed as a morally distasteful political system. In a similar vein, Nestlé food products became the focus of an international boycott by those opposed to the marketing of infant formula milks in developing countries. Although infant formula is a satisfactory alternative to breast milk where clean water and hygienic environmental conditions prevail it easily becomes a source of infection when polluted water and dirty feeding bottles are used. In addition, it is expensive for low-income rural dwellers to buy and while money needed for other things is spent on the prestigious 'formula', nutritionally and economically valuable breast milk is wasted. Costly formula is often diluted to make it last longer and thus becomes nutritionally unsatisfactory as well. The argument of the boycotters is not necessarily that there is something intrinsically wrong with formula milks, but that they are eminently unsuitable for use in the countryside and villages of the developing countries of the South. To actively promote them, as Nestlé and other companies do, is therefore at least unethical, if not downright immoral.

The Nestlé boycotters coordinated their protests by forming hundreds of action groups throughout the Northern world. They collected evidence, wrote letters and even published their own newsletters – all with a view to influencing company and government policy. Other food boycotts are not so high profile and may indeed operate simply at an individual level, having no discernable effect apart from that of quieting the conscience of the boycotter. For example, many large multinational food companies import raw foodstuffs from poor countries of the South. Such products as fruit, coffee and cacao command far higher prices when they reach the American and European markets than are paid to the primary producers. On foreign-owned plantations, local workers may be paid poverty-line wages to grow and harvest crops which will make huge corporate profits abroad. By refusing to buy the products of particular companies consumers in the affluent world make their own protest against exploitation and greed. Although they do not expect to be able to change the system they can at least decline to participate in one part of it.

Boycotts do of course have political and economic as well as moral implications. Many people would not consider joining a boycott because they would see it as being politically motivated and quite ineffective as a tool for change. However, practicality and efficiency are not generally the criteria used for making moral or ethical choices; more to the point is what is considered to be right or wrong.

Non-meat-eating

Vegetarianism as a style of eating may be the result of necessity, either economic or ecological, or of choice. As a matter of choice it can be freely practised on an individual basis or collectively adopted for religious or philosophical reasons.

From an economic point of view, meat is an expensive component of the traditional Western diet; the cost of the shopping basket can be considerably reduced if this class of foods is restricted or omitted. Normally, no nutritional harm results if suitable adjustments are made; for example, if consumption of fish and of dairy products is increased or if cereals, nuts and pulses are used as protein sources. It was once common for nutritionists and dietitians to exhort their clients, particularly the poor and the elderly, to substitute less expensive cuts of meat for prime cuts as a way of saving money. Although seemingly rational from both an economic and nutritional point of view, this advice entirely ignores psychological effects on esteem and status. Meat is usually considered to be a high-status food and its forced disappearance from the table, in quantity or quality, has negative connotations. There is no doubt though that meat consumption does decline to some extent when household economics dictates cuts in food expenditures.

In many parts of the world meat is simply not available, at least in other than very small quantities; diets consist largely of cereal or starchy root staples. Under these circumstances vegetarianism is a condition imposed by the material environment; were meat to be readily available then it would be eaten.

For many others though, non-meat-eating is a personal or collective choice which reflects certain views about the world and the place of humans and animals in it. Eastern philosophies, as well as those of North American aboriginal peoples, emphasize the mutual dependence of people and their environment; human beings are part of the world and must live in harmony with the rest of creation. Hindu and Buddhist beliefs in metempsychosis, the transmigration of souls, disallow the taking of a life which, after all, may contain the soul of an ancestor or of a potential child. This reverence for life is most fully expressed by sects such as the Jains. In sharp contrast is the Judao–Christian view that Man was given dominance over the Earth and thus has the right to exploit world resources, including animals, for his own ends. Berman (1982), who acts sometimes as a critic, sometimes as an apologist, for meat-eating by Jews maintains that compassion toward animals is a major theme in the Bible and that meat-eating was only permitted by God after the Flood because that was what ordinary men wanted. It was thus a concession to man's imperfection; after two millennia, still we are not morally ready to forego the eating of flesh.

Vegetarianism as a tenet of religious faith has been more fully described in the preceding chapter. Whereas some religious practitioners are not entirely conscientious in following dictates concerning food avoidance, other individuals without particular religious beliefs deliberately eschew the use of meat for a variety of reasons. Some believe that a vegetarian diet is healthier for the body and they therefore adopt a simple pattern of eating which emphasizes the use of fruits, vegetables and whole cereals and pulses. Such a diet tends to be higher in bulk and lower in calories, sugars and fats than a typical meat-centred regime; thus it is not surprising that studies have found vegetarians to be lighter on average than non-vegetarians, and to have lower blood cholesterol levels and lower blood pressures. The role of enthusiasts such as Graham and Kellogg in promoting vegetarianism in the 19th century is discussed below. They were able to take advantage of the new scientific enlightenment to add arguments based on health to their moral armoury. Graham employed 'a Christianized science in which the laws of health were treated as a physical counterpart to the Ten Commandments'. (Whorton, 1994).

Another group of vegetarians avoid meat for ecological reasons; meat production is an energy-intensive process, particularly when it is carried out in large-scale feed-lots. Grain which could be used directly for human food is instead fed to cattle; in the process of converting grain to meat large amounts of food energy are wasted. The rising world demand for meat, epitomized by the meat-centred diet of North Americans, encourages the use of energy-intensive methods of food production. In US feed lots grain is fed to cattle with a tenfold loss of energy. Battery hens utilize 5–10 lb grain per hen to produce 1 lb of meat or eggs. One pound of pork that provides 1000–2000 kcal at the table takes 14 000 kcal to produce and requires 1628 l of water (Durning and Brough, 1991). According to Rifkin (1992) there are a billion and a quarter cattle on earth, occupying a quarter of the planet's land mass and consuming enough grain to feed hundreds of millions of people. In the conversion of rainforest to pasture for cattle raising (55 square feet of rainforest per pound of hamburger) bird, animal and plant species are destroyed. Some 70% of the grain produced in the US is used to feed cattle and other livestock and the production of this grain accounts for half the water consumed in that country. Statistics such as these prompt some authorities to claim that vegetarianism allows for a more equitable sharing of the world's resources. Gussow (1994) addresses the question of whether environmental responsibility demands the elimination of livestock. While she rejects as impractical, Rifkin's utopian vision of a return to a 'natural' world, she leaves little doubt that current methods of animal rearing are wasteful and unsustainable and should be eliminated. Instead, animal rearing should be re-integrated into traditional pastoralist practices where animals are part of the natural ecosystem, and are raised for food instead of primarily for profit.

Ethical vegetarians believe that it is wrong to kill or harm animals, though they do not necessarily subscribe to particular religious doctrines. Prior to the rise of science as a dominant force, the non-eating of animals was justified entirely with moral and metaphysical arguments against the cruel exploitation of animals and the value of vegetarianism in achieving an exalted spiritual state (Whorton, 1994). Contemporary arguments for the non-use of animals as human food are advanced by Peter Singer (1976, 1979), who suggests that animals have as much right to existence as do humans and that they are not merely means to human ends. Singer concludes that becoming a vegetarian is the most practical and effective step one can take toward ending both the killing of non-human animals and the infliction of suffering upon them.

There is an ambivalence in our attitude toward animals in that while we profess to love them we do not hesitate to kill them when it suits us to do so. Sometimes emotions can over-ride the impulse, as in the case of a favourite rabbit saved from the pot through a mixed sense of love and guilt. For the subsistence hunter there was a direct connection between the animal and the act of eating; although animals were killed they were also respected and often worshipped or given as offerings to the Gods. In modern societies where a complex food supply chain has replaced the direct hunter–animal relationship meat has become merely another convenience product to be bought at the retailers. The ultimate result is seen at the modern supermarket where pre-cut, plastic-wrapped, aseptic-looking products bear little resemblance to anything that was once an animal. Indeed this sense of animal as commodity is epitomized by modern methods of animal rearing on feed lots and in batteries where the animal is raised in the most cost-efficient manner, often under miserable conditions, expressly for the purpose of being slaughtered. It is difficult to see that there is any respect for life here.

Delicacy and aesthetic considerations may prompt the refusal of meat. The work of Elias was discussed earlier in relation to table manners. This same author interprets vegetarianism as a logical development in the civilizing process in which there is a strong tendency to remove the distasteful from the sight of society (Elias, 1978). He suggests that those who from more or less rationally disguised disgust at eating meat refuse it altogether are in the vanguard of a larger social movement. Though their 'threshold of repugnance' is lower than that of 20th century civilized standards as a whole, and they are therefore considered to be deviant by their contemporaries, they are following the same direction that has produced changes in the past. Whereas the carving of a dead animal at table was once entirely acceptable, nowadays any reminders that a meat dish has anything to do with the killing of an animal are avoided to the utmost. The rejection of meat altogether is the next logical step on this typical civilization curve. Berman too, though he writes from a religious perspective, associates meat eating with an earlier stage of human history and claims that vegetarianism is a better response to today's world. 'Vegetarianism is surely a foretaste of life on earth in generations ahead.' (Berman, 1982).

Finally, vegetarianism in one of its many forms may be adopted by social groups as part of a counter-culture identity. Sometimes these groups adopt a belief system which borders on or leads to cultist behaviour.

FOOD REFORM, CULTS AND QUACKERY

Until relatively recently, nutrition was indivisible from medicine. As the science of medicine developed over the last two centuries it gradually lost interest in nutrition; faith in treatment and cure was transferred from food to drugs. While the medical profession gave up on nutrition, and the field was gradually colonized by a small and relatively powerless new professional corp of dietitians, faith in the power of nutrition remained strong among what Mowbray (1992) calls the **food reformers** – those who believe there is a perfect dietary regimen to prevent every ill and achieve disease-free and lengthy lifespans. Some, less kind, would call them quacks and there are certainly plenty of examples of unscrupulous practice. It seems that some people have always been concerned about what others eat and eager to comment on and attempt to influence those choices. There is a moralistic dimension to this desire which transcends the physiological value, real or supposed, of dietary exhortations. Many dietary philosophies are presented in the context of a total way of life, and some of these, such as macrobiotics, discussed below, attain the status of cults.

History

Food reform has a long history, the modern movement drawing heavily on pre-scientific ideas to re-establish the intimate connection between food and medicine. It emerged strongly during the 19th century through the work of people like Sylvester Graham, and is based on a handful of presumptions or principles which support the primacy of diet in achieving and maintaining health. Almost everyone is sick and almost everyone eats poorly; there are good foods and bad foods; everyone is responsible for improving their health through proper selection of diet. Mowbray comments that 'A rich mix of faith in diet, nature and moral law, with hosannahs to science and hostility to establishment medicine was in fact the recipe for the food and health reform books of the twentieth century'. This heady mix formed the basis of the search for perfect dietary regimens which continues today.

Food reformers have always had a pre-occupation with a 'natural diet'. To call a food natural is to call it good. In the 1830s in the US, a Presbyterian preacher named Sylvester Graham proclaimed vegetarianism to be the natural diet. 'Fruits, nuts, farinaceous seeds and roots, with perhaps some milk and it may be honey, in all rational probability constituted the food of the first family and the first generations of mankind.' (Graham, 1883, cited in Young 1970). Meat and fat were bad because they heated the temper and led to sexual excess. (Note the resemblance of this to the humoural theory of the ancient world.) Mustard, catsup and pepper could cause insanity. White bread was bad but bread made from coarse unsifted flour was good, provided it was slightly stale and had bran in it, as bran was good for regularity. Graham's teachings were quickly taken up; Graham hotels opened, operating on his espoused principles, and Grahamites adhered faithfully to their leader's dietary strictures. As his fame spread, Graham became more and more outrageous with his claims for the virtues of a vegetarian diet. But although his dietary ideas were somewhat bizarre and often taken to excess, Graham did awaken an interest in the health value of foods and at the same time set the pattern for future food reformers. During his lifetime he did not profit personally through the sale of his health food products or through his writings; his name is now remembered because it is used widely in the breakfast food industry.

The case of Dr. Kellogg has already been mentioned (cf. Seventh Day Adventism). His famous cornflakes were at first known as 'Elijah's manna' and were admired for their technological, and hence spiritual, purity. Kellogg, and his competitors, in effect translated Graham's radical dietary prescription into a mainstream mass-marketable convenience food offering; or as Mowbray puts it, health in a box.

Contemporary food reform

Reform themes from the 19th century persist into the 20th. Modern food reform has revived the notion of 'food as medicine' as one of its fundamental appeals. Contemporary food fads usually fall into one of three categories: (i) those in which the virtue of a particular food or food component are exaggerated and purported to cure specific diseases (e.g. garlic, lecithin); (ii) those advocating omission of certain foods because of harmful properties ascribed to them (e.g. white bread, sugar); and (iii) those emphasizing 'natural foods'. Reformist claims raise doubts about the purity of the ordinary food supply, and create a market for the special products sold by the health food stores.

Advocates of food reform employ a number of common strategies for promoting their views. They offer stories of personal cure and salvation, they bolster their own credibility by simply asserting that they are knowledgeable and fudge or ignore dates so as to make old ideas seem contemporary.

Mowbray (1992) adds that arguments are often contradictory and internally inconsistent, so: 'Drug therapy is condemned, but drug-like effects are claimed for vitamins, minerals, amino acids and other constituents of food. The authority of the medical profession is challenged, but professional credentials (sometimes in unrelated fields and from diploma mills) are used to establish authority. Scientists are condemned for ignoring important facts but scientific experiments are freely quoted when they seem to support an unorthodox position. There is a general hunger for scientific validation'.

In the face of this populist movement, orthodox nutrition and medicine is quick to react – some would say over-react – to condemn what is regarded as quackery. The scientific establishment has little sympathy for differing beliefs or experiences and many professionals would rather ridicule lay practices than try to understand them. Nevertheless, outright quackery and fraud does exist to the detriment of both health and economic well-being. Dr. Victor Herbert provides pointers for recognizing the quack (Table 7.1) and attacks the multi-million dollar industry of quackery, revealing corruption, deception and brainwashing on a mammoth scale (Herbert, 1980).

Table 7.1 Sixteen tips to recognize the quack

1. He advises that you go out and buy something which you would not otherwise have bought.

2. He is a fake specialist with imposing 'front' titles. Use of Institute and Society titles which mean nothing.

3. He says that most disease is due to a bad or faulty diet.

4. He says that most people are poorly nourished (sub-clinical deficiency gambit).

5. He tells you that soils depletion and use of chemical fertilizers causes malnutrition.

6. He alleges that modern processing methods and storage remove all nutritive value from our food.

7. He tells you that you are under stress and that in certain diseases your need for nutrients is increased.

8. He says you are in danger of being poisoned by food additives and preservatives

9. He tells you that if you eat badly, you'll be OK if you take a vitamin or vitamin and mineral supplement (this is the 'nutrition insurance' gambit).

10. He recommends that everyone take vitamins or health foods or both.

11. He claims that natural vitamins are different from synthetic ones.

12. He promises quick, miraculous and dramatic cures.

13. He uses testimonials and case histories to support his claims

14. He'll offer you a vitamin that isn't (pangamate – Vit B15; laetrile – Vit B17)

15. He espouses the 'conspiracy theory' and its twin, the controversy claim. He says he is being persecuted and his work suppressed. Or that there is a controversy between himself and orthodoxy.

16. He is legally belligerent. If a nutritionist travels with a lawyer and threatens libel actions against those who disagree with him, he is probably a quack.

Reprinted with permission from, Herbert V. (1980) *Nutrition Cultism*, G.F. Stickley Co. Philadelphia.

Reasons for food faddism

There is no doubt that thousands of people unthinkingly become victims of food faddism through misconceptions about the nature of food and diet. Wang (1971) defined a misconception as 'a belief commonly held as true but which is not in accord with scientific evidence'. But as we have seen above, science is not the yardstick by which food reformers and food faddists operate. Social psychologists as well as nutritionists have studied the phenomenon of food faddism and have offered a number of explanations for its persistence.

The search for good health, personal beauty and perpetual youth has always been an alluring goal. Modern Western society, as mirrored in its popular culture, glorifies youthfulness and thinness. Commercial interests offer thousands of products to aid in the fight to remain young and trim. As this or that food supplement, dieting scheme or herbal extract is promoted there are strong cultural pressures to follow the trend, particularly where the influence of peers is important. For this reason, teenagers may be especially prone to food fads.

One of the greatest commodities that food faddists have to offer is hope. Although their promises may be unrealistic – or even bizarre – when all else fails in confronting serious illness there is always the chance that a miracle herb or food will do the trick. The faith placed in such cures may indeed lead to subjective feelings of enhanced well-being and thus be of real benefit to the user. All too often though there are potentially harmful side effects associated with the use of dietary supplements and adjuncts.

The opposite side of the coin to hope, is fear. For people who are anxious about their health, faddist prescriptions offer a defence against the threats supposedly posed by modern living. Vague aches and pains for which orthodox medicine offers no diagnosis or remedies may be kept at bay by exotic dietary nostrums. Although this may be interpreted as a form of hypochondriasis it may also be seen as an attempt by people to improve their own health. Kandel and Pelto (1980) suggest that the health food movement could be viewed as a process of social revitalization and as an alternative health maintenance system which emphasizes prevention rather than cure.

As in the case of vegetarianism discussed earlier, faddist dietary practices can serve as a form of personal and group expression of identity. They signal mistrust of orthodox medicine and of modern agriculture and represent a sort of anti-establishment lifestyle. Faddists frequently perceive an unholy alliance between scientists, government and the food industry who are conspiring to rob them of their health, though they seem to ignore a similar alliance between health food promoters, food supplement companies and unorthodox educational establishments. Oddly enough, many of the people who criticize the artificiality of the food supply and who abhor the use of additives are the same people who willingly swallow a multitude of dietary supplements in the form of pills, powders and potions.

As De Garine (1970) has said, in many cases the judgements made by orthodox practitioners on food cults and fads are nothing more than value judgements which describe the faddist behaviour as deviating from the modern concept of food as reduced to its nutritional, economic and organoleptic properties. Thus while it is possible to discount food faddism as being merely the result of ignorance, gullibility and exploitation, it is also possible to see in it a legitimate attempt by individuals to pursue good health and peace of mind. A good example of how this quest can lead beyond diet to a total way of life is discussed below.

Macrobiotics

Adherents claim that macrobiotic principles have been recognized for centuries as the key to good health and longevity. The term was first used in the literature in 1796 by Von Hufeland, a German physician. In modern times it has been developed as a dietary and spiritual regime based on the principle that a wholesome diet is the most direct path to good health. George Ohsawa, born Yukikazu Sakurazawa, reputedly cured himself of serious illnesses by adopting a simple diet based on brown rice, miso soup and vegetables. Coming to Europe in the 1920s he devoted the rest of his life to writing and teaching about macrobiotics. A macrobiotic diet is said to offer spiritual enlightenment through a combination of mental discipline and ascetic eating habits.

Table 7.2 Macrobiotics: the yin–yang general classification

Yang
      Poultry
      Eggs
      Cheese
      Beef
      Fish
      Cereal grains
      Milk
      Beans
      Pork
      Root vegetables
      Leafy vegetables
      Seeds
      Nuts
      Fruit
      Sugar
              Yin

In the modern practice of macrobiotics, principles of yin and yang have been applied to a vegetarian-style diet in which brown rice and miso soup are the main components. Yin and yang represent the opposing forces of the universe, which are also present within individuals. Foods are placed on a continuum ranging from extreme yin foods like sugar to extreme yang products such as meat and eggs (Table 7.2), though it is important to recognize that yin and yang are relational attributes; that is, fruit is not by definition yin, but is only yin in comparison to something which is more yang such as eggs. Dairy products are difficult to classify as yin or yang because some, such as goat and sheep products are very yang while others such as cream and yoghurt are very yin. Categories of foods thus vary internally in their degree of yin or yang, and so do individual foods. One carrot may be more yin than another. This is a reflection of one of Ohsawa's Seven Laws of the Order of the Universe, that of non-identity. Directly opposing the scientific belief that, say, all carbohydrates are the same if their chemical composition is the same, macrobiotics holds that all carbohydrates are different and this has important influences on the macrobiotic diet where the skilled practitioner chooses between more or less yin or yang produce (Aihara, 1985). Differences in apparently identical foods arise because their degree of yin or yang is influenced by many factors including their origin, species, season and method of growing, cooking and way of storage. Whole-grain cereals and vegetables are in the centre of the yin–yang continuum and thus are most appropriate in bringing about a harmonious condition in the body. (cf. Allopathy). Dairy products, meat, sugar and alcohol should be avoided, while fruit intake should be restricted. Foods are also divided into acid- and alkaline-forming categories, which must be balanced. Proportions of food in a basic macrobiotic diet then looks something like Figure 7.1.

The rationale given for macrobiotic practices is a mixture of appeals to history, to what people have 'traditionally' eaten, to philosophy and spirituality and to the unhealthy state of the modern food supply. Meat, for example, should be avoided because it is rich in fat, because its breakdown in the body causes build up of harmful wastes, because of the chemical additives and antibiotics used in raising animals, and because of the factory farm conditions in which animals are raised. Sometimes, even the generally reviled Western science is embraced. Macrobiotics had no explanation based on nutritional or physiological principles for its recommendation of a grain-based diet, but it enthusiastically embraced the Dietary Goals report of the Select Senate Committee on Nutrition and Human Needs (1977) which recommended that 55–60% of total energy intake should be derived from complex carbohydrate. Contemporary exponents of macrobiotics point to the congruence between it and orthodox dietary goals in elevating the importance of whole-grain cereals and reducing fat intake. For example, Kushi (1985) says that the transition to a macrobiotic diet should be a gradual one beginning by reducing the

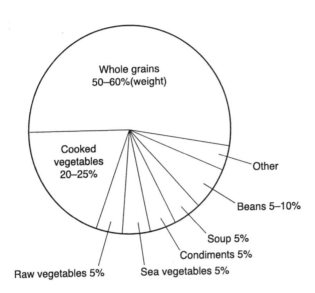

Figure 7.1 Composition of the macrobiotic diet. (A certain latitude exists among the proportions of component foodstuffs allowed; hence the dietary total may appear to exceed 100%)

amount of saturated fats, refined starches and sugars in the diet. Whole grains, vegetables and beans should be eaten more frequently. Food should be grown locally and consumed in as natural state as possible.

The diet first achieved notoriety when a young woman starved to death on a brown rice diet during her effort to reach a state of enlightenment. Like other vegetarian regimes, macrobiotic diets can meet nutritional needs, but may become too restrictive if focused solely on grains. Strict adherence to the more rigid diets can result in scurvy, anaemia and hypoproteinaemia, hypocalcaemia and ultimately, death. Calorie intake is usually low, and poor growth is the main clinical finding in infancy. A report of two infants fed on kokkoh (a macrobiotic food mixture for infants, consisting of a mixture of brown rice, wheat, oats, sesame seeds and beans) from birth to 7 and 14 months respectively, showed that they were substantially underweight and short in length (Robson *et al.*, 1974). Others have claimed that the benefits of the macrobiotic diet include normalized blood pressure and low serum levels of cholesterol, and that reports of malnutrition are either based on inadequate evidence, are due to misapplication of the dietary principles or are isolated cases. However, a population study which included 80% of the macrobiotic children in the

Netherlands clearly demonstrated widespread deficiencies of energy, protein, vitamin B-12, vitamin D, calcium and riboflavin leading to growth retardation, muscle wasting and slower psychomotor development (Dagnelie and van Staveren, 1994).

The goal of macrobiotics is to make everyone rich and 'to live a long, amusing, happy life, realizing one's dreams one by one' (Aihara, 1985). Other goals include freedom from financial worries (achieved through a simple lifestyle) and the development of supreme judgement. Attainment of such judgement, which allows one to see that all antagonisms are complementary, will lead to resolution of all worldly problems. The final goal of macrobiotics is nothing less than world peace. Once again, we see that nutrition is intimately entwined with philosophical ideas; diet is a means to a moral end.

The prudent diet

While busy challenging the legitimacy of non-scientific approaches to health and nutrition, the nutrition establishment may have invented its own version of the enduring dietary regimen in the form of the **prudent** diet. In Chapter 2 we saw how post-war prosperity in North America shifted nutrition concerns from ones of insufficiency to ones of over-sufficiency. The question arose as to whether the nation's diet should be drastically modified, and nutrition policy became more important than nutrition science. 'Nutrition had found an agenda of great interest to the well-off and the well-fed; it had become politicized' (Mowbray, 1992).

Guides on correct diet appeared with increasing frequency until 'The 1980s would develop into the most nutrition-obsessed decade so far in the twentieth century, with much of the obsession focused on a key reform idea – that chronic and degenerative diseases such as cancer and heart disease were a plague upon the land, were caused by poor diet, and could be prevented and sometimes cured by regimen' (Mowbray, 1992). Food reformers and prudent diet enthusiasts had found common cause, even if they continued to offer different solutions.

The relative lack of strong evidence has not stopped calls for major changes in the diet of industrialized countries. 'At its worst, prudent diet enthusiasm yields all the absurd and tiresome side effects of any reform enthusiasm: intense response by food marketers and manufacturers - silly products, distorted health claims, shrill, quick-cure books and articles, disapproving looks and moralizing comments of people who do not like the way other people eat'. (Mowbray, 1992).

Just as the followers of macrobiotic regimens produce health problems for themselves or their offspring so can the devotees of prudent diet regimens run into difficulties. Parents may have exaggerated concerns about excessive food intake by their children and may worry unduly about the development of obesity and atherosclerosis. Pugliese *et al.* (1987) describe cases where such parental beliefs led to parents putting their children on diets currently in vogue and approved by the medical community for adults who are at risk for cardiovascular disease, with the result that infants experienced inadequate weight gain and decreased linear growth. Mowbray suggests that the current obsession with nutrition is not healthy and that nutrition science, at the end of the century of its great triumph, risks being cast into the service of hypochondria, unrealistic expectations, and displacement activity.

SUMMARY

Religious belief is not the only basis for moral or ethical food practices. Vegetarianism is practised by diverse communities for reasons which include respect for life, conservation of the environment and equitable distribution of scarce resources.

Cultism is a term used to describe patterns of eating which are, in terms of conventional nutritional wisdom, bizarre. Cultism may be centred around the supposed efficacy of one particular dietary substance or may involve quite complex patterns of food behaviour. A cult often assumes a pseudo-religious mantle among its followers, and indeed has some common ground with orthodox religions in that faith is usually a strong characteristic of its adherents. The tendency of some nutritionists to merely dismiss food cultists as ignorant and dangerous fanatics is a misguided one. Cultist food practices undoubtedly answer social and psychological needs in their practitioners in much the same way as do orthodox food practices for non-cultists. That the foods chosen are unusual or nutritionally undesirable does not make the reasons for their use any less important to understand. Unfortunately though, whereas a questionable nutritional practice may be tolerated because it is religiously inspired, the same practice is often derided if it is perceived to be a consequence of cultism.

FURTHER READING

Macrobiotics as a way of life is described in Aihara (1985), while Kushi (1985) provides a basic introduction to the principles plus practical information on recipes and food preparation.

For a comprehensive overview of historical, moral, ecological, nutritional and practical dimensions of vegetarianism see the 24 contributed papers in Johnston, P.K. (ed.) (1994) Second International Congress on Vegetarian Nutrition, *Am. J. Clin. Nutr.*, **59**(suppl).

Mowbray (1992) is a thought-provoking and entertaining guide to the topic of food reform through the ages.

DISCUSSION QUESTIONS

1. Is vegetarianism for all a viable way of: (i) conserving world food resources; (ii) alleviating world hunger?
2. To what extent does the fact that moral statements about non-animal eating are culturally specific affect their strength? Are cultures which do not share such values immoral?
3. Discuss the cases of sugar and cholesterol in the context of faddism.
4. Are the users of health foods and nutritional supplements victims of fraud and self-deception or are they in the vanguard of health promotion by taking control over their own health and well-being?

CHAPTER 8

Myths, taboos and superstitions

A myth is a traditional narrative, usually involving supernatural or fancied persons, and embodying popular ideas on natural or social phenomena. Malinowski (1963) saw myths as being in the nature of charters; that is, stories of the first doing of an act that are still repeated in ritual or that validate some claim in social relationships. They explain why what is done today is the right thing to do. Sacredness and ritual are characteristics of myth and may be combined with elements of legends or fairy-tales. Legends recount supposed history whereas fairy-tales deal with miraculous happenings which no-one supposes to be true and which are pure entertainment. It may be that myths also serve to explain and impose order on the incomprehensible universe (Freidl and Pfeiffer, 1977).

Modern science is a means of embodying ideas about natural phenomena, based on observable facts rather than on supernatural beliefs; but because observations are subjective in nature and thus are often incomplete, if not actually erroneous, it is possible that nutritional doctrine accepted today may contain unseen errors which, being reified, pass into the mythology of dietary dogma. However, at least in principle, science is to be questioned and changed if the facts dictate change; myth is essentially religious or sacred and is thus not questionable.

FOOD AND MAGIC

Sir George Frazer expressed the early view that magic was a sort of pseudo-science, preceding genuine science. Malinowski (1963) pointed out that it is highly unlikely that magical beliefs would have been generally applied as an explanation of natural phenomena, for if people thought that like affected like all the time then they would become hopelessly confused by what actually happened in the real world. He maintained that science arose from the human ability to organize knowledge, whereas magic dealt with the organization of supernatural realities. Rather than being a way of interpreting the world in general magic is directed toward a specific end and involves manipulation of an object, albeit it in a supernatural manner. It is thus essentially pragmatic, seeking to gain control over forces in the Universe which cannot be understood in any other way.

Frazer, in his classic book, *The Golden Bough*, suggests that fundamentally there are two types of magic, sympathetic or homeopathic, and contact or contagious. In the first case, similar things can be considered the same. Magic effects can be achieved by working magic on an object which resembles or has the properties of the target selected. The ancient Doctrine of Signatures attributed properties to foods on the basis of their appearance; red beet juice was a cure for anaemia; yellow celandine a cure for jaundice. In the second case, actual contact with the object is required; contagious magic relies on touching or possessing part of the object or its belongings. Thus a hunter may perform magic on the spoor of an antelope in order to catch the beast itself. In addition, undesired effects can be avoided by avoiding contact with sympathetic objects, a case of negative magic. This, suggests Frazer, is the origin of taboo; an avoidance of what it is believed could cause harm. Ideas of sympathetic and contagious magic abound in food taboos. Thus snails and jackals are avoided by hunters who don't want to become cowardly and weak. Lions, and hearts of predators may be eaten to confer strength and courage. In parts of Nigeria it is believed that if children are reared on expensive foods then they will expect them when they are older, and will steal to get them (Ogbeide, 1974).

Practices based on sympathetic magic have also been reported from the Appalachian region of the US. Red beets are believed to cure low blood pressure, while to cure yellow jaundice 'break an egg, take the white and put it in a sack and hang it around the neck. They say the egg white will turn yellow' (Shifflett, 1976). In Britain, lactating women may be given milk stout to stimulate their own milk production. A modern example of sympathetic magical thinking in the world of commerce is to be found in the case of formula milks which strive to imitate breast milk.

For the Wamirans of Papua New Guinea, magic is what makes their staple crop, taro, grow. Failure of a taro crop is attributed to either the ritual incompetence of the cultivator or to sorcery on the part of an enemy. Each stage of cultivation is accompanied by magic, which is gender-related. Men possess magic for taro planing, women possess magic for weeding and tending the growing tubers. There is a strong taboo against being the first to eat one's own food. Ancestral spirits, konaga, live in the taro and reward an individual who properly observes custom with strong, heavy tubers as well as with personal health and well-being (Kahn, 1986).

Folklore and old wives' tales

Many foods are endowed with magical properties and beliefs in their efficacy are firmly held. Any rationalization for such beliefs recedes into the background with the passage of time, and the beliefs themselves become part of the conventional wisdom of the society to be passed down the generations in the form of folklore or, more pejoratively, old wives' tales. A wealth of traditional wisdom is bought to bear on weather prediction, birth rites and on food practices. Country cures, often involving the use of tisanes, are eagerly adopted by the children of science as though their very antiquity confers on them certain power. Whereas it is true that there is a strong empirical basis to support many practices, others rely on the kind of non-scientific rationalizations described above. For example, fish is widely touted as being a 'brain food'; in P.G. Wodehouse's timeless stories, Bertie Wooster is forever advising the inimitable Jeeves to eat fish in order to come up with a brainy scheme or ruse (see for example, Wodehouse, 1957). As it happens, fish is a good source of dietary potassium and potassium is indeed found in significant quantities in brain cells. The imaginative leap which is taken to ascribe a cause and effect relationship between eating fish and mental prowess is entirely fanciful. Does the belief that crusts will make hair curly have similar pseudo-scientific origins? Bringeus (1975) provides an account of Swedish folk beliefs surrounding the boiling of blood sausage. Silence is required during the process for when the lips are sealed the sausage skin will remain sealed also. Traditions which held that the sausage would burst its casing if a stranger came in probably derived rationally from the fact that draughts could blow the fire and cause uneven cooking.

In traditional Appalachian culture non-nutritional uses of food may be classified as occult, as in the example of eggs given above, or non-occult. Non-occult uses mainly take the form of household remedies in which food is used in a non-nutritional manner. These remedies are handed down over many generations, sometimes in writing but often orally, and frequently pertain to poultices made of food and to the use of food in pain relief. For fever 'take a grated potato – salt it down heavy and put it on the forehead'. For rheumatism 'rub mustard and beet leaves on the pained part; tie it on with a cloth' (Shifflett and Nyberg, 1978). In a Californian investigation, Newman (1969) found that the recitation of folk beliefs to a primiparous woman symbolized her entry into the new estate of motherhood.

PROHIBITIONS AND TABOOS

Whereas magical thinking leading to the avoidance of certain items can explain the basis of many food practices and taboos it is only one of several factors contributing to varied and elaborate systems of prohibitions found throughout the world (Table 8.1). A belief basic to all religions, modern or primitive, is the attribution of a spirit or soul to living things. This belief is known as animism, and inherent in it is the worship of some spirit which is thought to have supernatural power and which may be either animate or inanimate. The Melanesians called this power mana, and it could be a source of both danger and beneficence. Food is loaded with power, or mana, which affects its suitability for consumption by certain individuals and at particular times of the year. Taboo is a restriction on human behaviour to avoid contact with mana. This, according to de Garine (1970), is the basis of many prohibition systems. The same author provides us with a schema to classify prohibitions (Table 8.2).

Table 8.1 Reasons for food taboos and avoidances

Disgust – fear of contamination
Unfamiliarity
Intimate familiarity
Fear of infertility
Condition of flesh – decayed, diseased
Hygiene – health
To restrict slaughter of useful animals
Sympathetic magic
Transmigration of souls
Totemism
Sacredness of animal
Religious sanctions
Cultural identity

Table 8.2 Classification of food prohibitions

According to their length
  (i)   Temporary prohibitions
  (ii) Permanent prohibitions
According to the size of human group they interest
  (i)   A number of societies
  (ii)   A total society
  (iii) One of the kinship groups in a given society
  (iv)   A socioprofessional group
  (v)   A social class
  (vi)   A masculine or feminine part of the society
  (vii) Individuals according to specific individual experiences
Temporary avoidances
  (i)   Pregnant and lactating women
  (ii)   Infant until weaning
  (iii) Baby during weaning
  (iv)   Infancy
  (v)   Puberty and adolescence
  (vi)   Sickness ... material or psychic

Adapted from De Garine, I. (1970) The Social and Cultural Background of Food Habits in Developing Countries (Traditional Societies), in *Symposium on Food Cultism and Nutritional Quackery*, (ed. G. Blix), Swedish Nutrition Foundation, Almqvist and Wiksells, Uppsala.

Taboos maintain the discreteness of categories but at the same time are ambiguous and thus a source of conflict and tension. They therefore become sacred, unmentionable, intriguing, dangerous and powerful (Leach, 1976). The concept of taboo should be carefully distinguished from that of simple avoidance, which is usually based on empirical common sense. Let us say, for example, that eating a particular berry always causes vomiting; after sufficient trials to establish the cause-and-effect relationship, that berry will be henceforth avoided; if, however, it is believed that eating over-ripe bananas during pregnancy causes brown spots on the skin of the baby, the supposed relationship is a magic or supernatural one and may lead to the establishment of a taboo to avoid the supposed danger. There are also plenty of examples of inverse taboos, where only certain groups of the society are allowed to consume particular foods. Most permanent taboos and avoidances have little effect on the nutrition of the individual practising them. However, temporary avoidances affect individuals at certain crucial periods of their life cycles and can have a very adverse effect. Ogbeide (1974) showed that in mid-west Nigeria the animal protein intake of children and of pregnant women was directly and adversely influenced by food taboos and avoidances. The temporary food avoidances of pregnant Tamilnad women are based on a fear of abortion. Papaya, which because of its shape may symbolize the female breast, and sesame are commonly avoided (Ferro-Luzzi, 1974). After a woman has given birth there is a 41-day pollution period during which impure foods are restricted (Table 8.3). A similar 40-day laying-in period is prescribed for Malay women, who avoid 'cold' fruit and vegetables, and 'toxic' fish (Wilson, 1973).

Table 8.3 Food avoidances amongst women of Tamilnad

Food	Avoidance period	Food	Avoidance period
'cold' foods	C	'hot' foods	C
meat in general	ABCD	chicken	ACD
chicken eggs	ABCD	sardines	D
crabs	C	cow's milk	ABCD
butter	ABD	fruits in general	D
all vegetables	C	potato	CD
in quantity		yam	D
rice	CD	millet	A
dhals	ACD	cashew nuts	D
chillies	ABCD	onion	D
pickles in general	A	salt	A

A = puberty: B = menstruation: C = pregnancy:
D = puerperium & lactation

Source: Adapted from Ferro-Luzzi G.E. (1974) Food Avoidances during the puerperium and lactation in Tamilnad, *Ecol.Food & Nutr.*, 3:7-15. With permission of Gordon and Breach Science Publishers.

Food avoidances and taboos can have the function of introducing social status differences between individuals and social groupings and of assigning people their place in society. Widespread prohibitions applied to women against the eating of flesh foods may have partly been derived from the male wish to keep the foods for themselves (Trant, 1954). Bolton (1972) reports that the aboriginal Orang Asli in West Malaysia taboo many animal proteins, especially to women of childbearing age and to children. Some foods are thought to contain spirits which may harm those who eat them; other animals are rejected because they have a special relationship to humans: they are 'kindred spirits'. Jelliffe and Jelliffe (1978) suggest that the reservation of the best foods for males reflects the ancient situation where it was imperative that the hunters be well fed. Such male privileging continues today (cf. Gender).

The Gitksan Indians of British Columbia forbade fresh meat to young girls during seclusion times at puberty and to all women during menstruation; breaking of this prohibition would bring bad luck to the family in all they did. Young boys were forbidden to eat certain parts of animals such as the head and legs of the bear, and pregnant women faced many restrictions regarding meat. Even today people would not want to spoil the hunting season by giving away meat to a woman who shouldn't it eat (People of 'Ksan, 1980).

Flesh taboos

Most food taboos are of flesh foods and they are often held with the strongest of convictions. The Sepoy rebellion of 1857 was sparked by the insensitiveness of British military officers who issued rifle cartridges which were greased with pork and cattle fat to Hindu and Moslem soldiers. The sepoys would not bite these cartridges as was necessary to uncap them. Taboos against pork consumption have already been discussed in Chapter 6 while avoidance of beef-eating is treated in detail in the following section on the Sacred Cow. Both of these taboos are relatively well known; the avoidance of eggs and chickens is less well appreciated though it is indeed widespread.

Simoons (1961) suggests that the avoidance arose in the Orient though it is now most common in Africa. Originally chickens were used for divination purposes and this role was only later usurped by their food potential. Many groups have associated eggs with fertility, childbirth and sex. Most aboriginal Malays do not eat eggs because of fertility beliefs. Religious beliefs attached to Hinduism and Buddhism have also fostered chicken and egg avoidance. Hindus may have avoided these foods to distinguish themselves from Moslems and from aboriginal tribes, because of their vegetarian beliefs, or because chickens were seen to be unclean. In

Buddhist India the prohibition is not strongly adhered to but in Tibet neither eggs nor chickens are widely used. Chickens are viewed as being unclean because of their dietary habits, and eggs are unclean because they come from fowl. Simoons gives numerous examples of egg avoidance in Africa showing that in some areas breaking of the taboo is merely disapproved of while in others it is severely sanctioned. The prohibition is sometimes applied to a whole group, sometimes only to individuals within that group – commonly women of childbearing age. Such restrictions are based on fear of barrenness, lasciviousness or of injury to the unborn child. In the Caribbean it is believed that eggs will make the foetus too big and that the baby will cry like a fowl. Also, that because eggs increase fertility, they can cause a child to become pregnant (Hope, 1975).

Horseflesh is tabooed not only in most of Europe and the New World but in many parts of the Old World too. Nevertheless, horsemeat was consumed with relish by humans in the early post-glacial period. Historically, horseflesh was eaten in northern Europe until the practice was suppressed by the spread of Christianity as described earlier. From a taboo with religious and sentimental connotations there evolved the notion that horsemeat was intrinsically unclean and then unhealthy (Gade, 1976). However, the practice never fully died out and there are historical reports indicating that horse-eating continued through the Middle Ages in Ireland, Denmark and Switzerland. In general though it became a low-status food and was largely avoided until the 18th century when widespread starvation conditions in France spurred a revival in its popularity. Horsemeat was popularized in France and Germany through banquets and specialist butcher shops and it gained a small degree of acceptance in both continental Europe and in Britain. Gade estimates that about one-third of modern Frenchmen eat some horse meat, though the practice is largely urban centred and working-class oriented. This author suggests that consumption has probably reached its peak due to a combination of residual social disapproval and cost which limits availability. However, it is one of the few examples of an attitude change from aversion to qualified approval. Simoons comments that even this limited attempt at countering a food prejudice was only possible when religion was no longer involved in the matter. As for the Old World situation, in areas such as the Mediterranean Basin where the horse was a luxury animal, eating those animals was ecologically undesirable. Buddha outlawed the eating of horseflesh and though Mohammed made no definite pronouncements most modern Moslems do not eat horseflesh. Others in Central Asia continue to do so. In India today horseflesh is eaten by some lower caste groups and it is quite acceptable to the Ainu of Japan. Argentina is the leading exporter of horsemeat, half of it going to Japan for use in sukiyaki and in sausages (Gade, 1976), while Canada is the major supplier to France.

Pariser and Hammerle (1966) draw attention to the widespread avoidance of fish as food, citing the dangerous nature of fishing, the sacredness of water and the perishability of fish itself as contributing factors. Fish is avoided in much of Asia, Africa and the South-West United States (cf. Hinduism).

Western taboos

Much of the literature concerning prohibitions and taboos relates to traditional or non-Western societies. It is true though, that Westerners hold equally irrational ideas regarding what is fit to be eaten. Because English Christians, say, do not eat insects or dogs or horses they tend to see these practices as being deviant or abhorrent; however, they will willingly eat the pig flesh which is forcefully rejected by Moslems and Jews. In his examination of dog-eating, Simoons sagely remarks that Western anthropologists rarely comment on dog-flesh avoidance because it is a prejudice which they themselves share. Avoidance in this instance is probably related to ideas of the dog as companion and friend, the so-called 'rover complex'. Obviously, no such qualms exist in mainland China, as shown by a report from the *London Times* of January 3rd, 1980.

> Peking, Jan 3 – A restaurant in Jilin, north-east China, was praised by the People's Daily for capitalist-style enterprise in ensuring supplies of its most popular item – dogmeat. It appealed to people to bring in their own dogs to be eaten and it would buy them. The result: in under a month it bought 1,369 dogs – a year's supply.

A valiant attempt to change attitudes toward a food source was made by the Victorian Englishman, Vincent M. Holt, who posed the challenge: 'Why not eat insects?' (Holt, 1885). In building his case Holt cites the biblical precedent of Leviticus and historical evidence of other races enjoying insects. 'We pride ourselves upon our imitation of the Greeks and Romans in their arts; we treasure their dead languages; why not then take a useful hint from their tables? We imitate the savage nations in their use of numberless drugs, spices and condiments; why not go a step further?'. Holt praises the virtues of insects as food not only because he sees them as tasty delicacies (much better than raw oysters and scavenging unclean lobsters) but because they also offer a solution to food shortages in England. He even provides recipes such as this one for grasshoppers which he says is based on a Moroccan locust recipe. 'Having plucked off their heads, legs and wings, sprinkle them with pepper and salt and chopped parsley; fry in butter and add some vinegar.' Finally, he suggests menus which 'if unnaturally crowded with insect items, serve as an illustration of what is possible' (Table 8.4).

There are several million types of insect which, on the face of it, should provide a prodigious and accessible source of food. Indeed, the enduring prejudice against eating insects seems to be a phenomenon of modern Western society. Despite our sensibilities though, it is difficult to

Table 8.4 An insectivorous menu

Slug soup
Boiled cod with snail sauce
Wasp grubs fried in the comb
Moths sauteed in butter
Braized beef with caterpillars
New carrots with wireworm sauce
Gooseberry cream with sawflies
Devilled chafer grubs
Stag beetle larvae on toast

Based on Holt, V. (1885) *Why not eat Insects?* Classey, Middx.

avoid eating insects. Aphids on salad greens, fragments of beetles in flour, rice weevils in rice are all next to impossible to avoid. Canned tomato products commonly contain fruit flies, beetles and tomato hook worms. Even government regulations acknowledge that it is impossible to avoid insect contamination and set limits based on consumer acceptability (Table 8.5).

As Mr Holt pointed out to the Victorians, there is plenty of historical evidence that people have always eaten insects; today they are eaten around the world, though mostly in the tropics and in Asia where they are most abundant. They are sometimes eaten whole, but often have legs and wings removed. Usually fried or roasted, they are also added to soups and stews, cakes or bread, ground into paste or dried into meal. Some people eat them as dietary staples; others only in times of famine; others as gourmet items. Mostly, insects are collected from the wild (cf. Chapter 2); some are sold and bought at markets; occasionally, they are reared commercially for the table (Taylor, 1973).

While insects are by and large unacceptable in Western cultures as normal sources of food, they may be of value in hardship situations. Taylor recommends eating those fresh insects which birds and mammals eat, and offers guidelines for the hungry but timid survivor (Table 8.6).

Table 8.5 Extracts from Extraneous Material Guidelines that relate to the safety and cleanliness of food

Product: Method: Defects	n	c	m	M
Bakery products (no fruit/nuts)				
Method ExFLP-22				
Rodent hairs	3	1	1/225g	3/225g
Cheese (whole or grated)				
Method ExFLP-5 (total filth)				
Insect fragments (not mites)	3	1	4/225g	8/225g
mites (dead)	3	1	25/225g	34/225g
rodent hairs	3	1	1/225g	3/225g
other mammalian hairs (not human)	3	1	1/225g	3/225g
Coffee (ground roasted beans)				
Insect fragments	3	1	35/25g	60/25g
Mushrooms (canned, dried, fresh, frozen)				
Method ExFLP-17				
Maggots < 2.0mm	6	2	10/100g	20/100g
Maggots ≥ 2.0mm	6	2	0/100g	5/100g
Mites (dead):	6	2	20/100g	75/100g
Mould	6		average of 10% or less of decomposed mushrooms by weight	
Nematodes	6	0	0/100g	0/100g
Rice (white, brown)				
Method ExFLP-21 (white) ExFLP-1 (brown)				
Whole or equiv. whole forms of insects				
Insect fragments	3	1	25/100g	50/100g
Rodent hairs	3	2	0/100g	3/100g
Wheat flour (white)				
Method ExFLP–19				
pre-milling insect frags. ≤ 0.2mm	3	1	20/50g	50/50g
post-milling insect frags. > 0.2mm	3	1	10/50g	20/50g
Rodent hairs	3	2	0/50g	2/50g

n = number of sample units usually but not always selected at random from a lot and examined in order to satisfy the requirements of a particular acceptance plan used.

c = maximum allowable number of marginally acceptable sample units.

m = acceptable concentrations of microorganisms or amounts of extraneous material. In a 2-class plan, m separates sample units of acceptable and defective quality; in a 3-class plan, m separates sample units of acceptable quality from those of marginally acceptable quality

M = (only in a 3-class plan) unacceptable concentrations of microorganisms of amounts of extraneous material that indicate a (potential) health or injury hazard, imminent spoilage or gross insanitation; M separates sample units of marginally acceptable quality from those of defective quality.

Standards and guidelines can be applied only when the appropriate method of analysis is used.

Adapted from *Health Protection Branch Standards and Guidelines for Microbiological Safety and General Cleanliness of Food – An Overview.* Volume 1 Compendium of Analytical Methods, Health Canada, 1992. With permission of the Minister of Supply and Services Canada 1994.

Table 8.6 Safety tips for insect consumption

1. The insect should not produce any irritation when handled and should be free from putrefying odours.

2. A small portion held inside the lower lip for a few minutes   should not cause irritation nor produce a burning, acrid, bitter or soapy taste.

3. If it tastes good, a small well-chewed portion should not produce vomiting or diarrhoea within 8 hours.

Based on information in Taylor, R.L. (1973) *Butterflies in my Stomach: Insects in Human Nutrition*, Woodbridge Pr. Publ. Co., Santa Barbara.

FOOD, SEX AND SYMBOLISM

Hunger is seen as a basic drive for survival of the individual whereas sex is a basic drive for survival of the species. It might be expected that there are parallels and interactions between these fundamental activities. There are indeed some similarities between food and sexual taboos. In a Thai village ideas about proper human relations are pinned to rules about the edibility of animals. Great-grandchildren may not intermarry; buffaloes reared under the roof should not be sacrificed on behalf of a member of the same house. Livestock and women are not to be 'consumed' at home but are reared for exchange (Lindenbaum, 1977). The Massa of Cameroon have rituals which allow an immigrant to consume the food products of the community in which he has established himself. As soon as he is assimilated in this respect he develops a strong avoidance towards getting married within the group which has adopted him (de Garine, 1976). Among the Kandya of Sri Lanka, cooking food for a man and eating the food he provides, signifies marriage (Yalman, 1967). The woman who cooks a man's food is his sexual partner even though eating, as well as many other activities, is done mostly apart.

Pigs and taro are the central foods for Wamirans of Papua New Guinea. Pigs are symbols of female sexuality and are controlled and exchanged by men in ways which order social relationships. 'Unable to master women, men master pigs which serve as tangible, manipulable and composite symbols of the unharnessable characteristics of women' (Kahn, 1986). Taro production by males is symbolically equated to female reproduction. 'Whereas women are seen as reproducing society naturally by giving birth to children and perpetuating matrilineal groups, men reproduce society culturally in the cultivation and exchange of taro'.

Food and sex may also be related through symbolism, here illustrated by the example of eggs, which have commonly represented fertility and fecundity in many cultures throughout the world. The modern children's custom of hunting for chocolate Easter eggs is itself a remnant of fertility rites (Leach, 1972). In 17th-century France a bride, on entering her new home, broke an egg to assure her fecundity. In Morocco an egg is used in magic rites or in medicine to encourage female fecundity and male virility. Among the Tamilnad too, eggs are recommended for their strengthening and fertility-increasing powers (Ferro-Luzzi, 1974). Bride and groom exchange eggs after the wedding ceremony in Iran, and there is a Chinese custom of feeding eggs to a new mother to ensure that her fecundity continues. Eggs as a symbol of life-to-come may have led to their widespread use for divination purposes.

TABOOS – TWO EXAMPLES

The rest of this chapter is devoted to examination of two prominent food prohibitions. The case of the Sacred Cow of Hinduism is illustrative of a complex interaction of religious and philosophical belief with environmental pressures giving rise to a prohibition which elevates the tabooed animal to a symbol of an entire way of life. The account of cannibalism shows how a practice universally reviled as a mark of barbarism is continued on a symbolic level and how even the most strongly sanctioned prohibitions may be relaxed when human survival is threatened.

The Sacred Cow

India has an estimated 180 million cattle – approximately one-third of the total world cattle population (Lodrick, 1981). The slaughter of these beasts for human food is generally forbidden. While people starve to death, cattle wander freely about the streets untouched. Nutrition educators concerned with cross-cultural studies have frequently commented that traditional practices should not be interfered with unless they are overwhelmingly negative in their effects. The case of India's Sacred Cow provokes an intense debate between interventionists and laissez-faire nutritionists. The taboo is often cited as the supreme example of irrationality, and there is an ongoing debate as to whether it is fundamentally ideological or utilitarian in origin and effect. Does it have an overall negative or dysfunctional impact on Indian society or is it in fact a functionally positive practice?

In India the cow is an especially revered animal; it is a symbol of motherhood and fertility. Cow calendars, carvings and posters attest to its symbolic representation of health and abundance. Prayers are offered for sick cows and garlands are hung around the animals's necks on festival days. Cows wander at will through villages and towns; devout Hindus will touch a passing cow and then touch their own foreheads. Feeding cows brings great merit. There are even government-run homes for aged cows. Respect for cows has been incorporated in the guiding principles of the constitution of India. Brown (1957) presents a widely accepted account of the origins of cow sanctity. He says that there are five contributing factors:

- role of the cow in Vedic ritual
- literal interpretation of words for cow used figuratively in Veda
- Vedic prohibitions against doing harm to Brahmans' cows
- the ahimsa concept
- association of the cow with the Mother Goddess cult.

Alternative explanations have been proposed which draw on political and economic factors, such as countering the impact of Buddhism and Islam or as an attempt on the part of rising urban states to keep more animals for their own use (Diener, Nonini and Robkin, 1978). A detailed analysis of the Rigveda reveals 700 references to the cow, in ritual and mythological contexts far more often than in relation to economics (Srinivasan, 1979). Thus, the first explanation usually offered for the taboo is the religious one. The cow was created by Brahma on the same day as were the Brahmins and so is to be venerated above all others. 'All that kill cows rot in hell for as many years as there are hairs on the body of the cow.' say the early scriptures. The cow also immediately precedes the human in the reincarnation cycle, and thus should not be killed. If a cow dies either through deliberate killing or through neglect, the 'human-to-be' must return to the beginning of the reincarnation cycle and go through 87 forms before reaching the status of man again.

The earliest Vedas, the Hindu sacred texts from the second millennium BCE, prohibit the slaughter and consumption of cattle except by priests on important sacrificial and ceremonial occasions – at which time beef eating was in fact obligatory. The Aryans who invaded North-West India about 1500 BCE placed a high value upon the cow due to its many uses in providing food, drink, fuel and leather as well as its function as a draught animal (Srinivasan 1979), though oxen were sacrificed to the Gods. Early Hindus ate the flesh of cows at ceremonial feasts presided over by Brahmin priests who acted, in a sense, as agents of the new Aryan overlords. Harris (1974) speculates that with growth in population it would have become increasingly difficult for the priests to provide sufficient meat for all at redistributive feasts. Therefore meat-eating was gradually restricted to become the privilege of a select group, the Brahmins themselves. Buddhism and Jainism may have arisen partly as protests against such an elitist system. Certainly, the Buddhist concept of ahimsa, or non-violence, played a major part in the shift from sacrifice to avoidance, and the Brahmins gradually came to see it as their sacred duty to prevent the slaughter and consumption of domestic animals. Indeed the later Vedas began to contain contradictory passages, some permitting, some tabooing the slaughter of cattle. Many sacred cow passages were probably added by later priests.

Even in 250 BC when he made Buddhism the state religion of India, King Asoka did not outrightly forbid the killing of cows; but by the beginning of the Christian era a ban on cow slaughter had become widespread.

The Code of Manu prescribed penances for the slaughter of cattle, and by about the seventh century the situation was essentially the modern one (Simoons, 1961). Thus cow worship is a relatively recent development evolving with changes in religious ideas. The rise of Islam may also have helped to entrench cow sanctity as a mark of religious separateness. Some non-Hindu groups continued to eat beef and today slaughter of cows by Moslems is still a source of friction between religious groups, though many Moslems and Sikhs forego beef in deference to their Hindu neighbours. At the same time, some low-caste Hindus do eat beef despite the social stigma attached to that action.

Cultural ecologists suggest that practices which are maladaptive do not flourish and that it follows therefore that the cow-killing prohibition must have had some rational function. Farb and Armelagos (1980) point to a population increase in India two millennia ago which necessitated massive cultivation of land to provide food. Subsequent deforestation and erosion had fatal consequences; droughts became commonplace and domestic animals became harder to maintain. Only those domestic animals which were essential could be allowed to share the diminishing amount of available land, and cows were essential as a source of traction animals for working the land. Farmers who maintained their cows during times of natural disasters survived, while those who ate their cows lost their tools of production. Over the centuries more and more farmers avoided eating their cows until an unwritten taboo came into existence. Only later was the taboo codified by the priesthood. Thus religious sanctions forbade the villagers to kill the cattle which were needed for other purposes than as a supply of meat (Harris, 1965, 1974). In this view, the religious element is an effect rather than a cause of the prohibition.

This thesis is criticized by many scholars in the field. Simoons (1979) argues that the environmental degradation was induced through overgrazing; he says it does not make sense that farmers would ban slaughter and thus increase cattle numbers and thereby intensify pressures on the environment. He also cites evidence from early literature which indicates that cow sanctity was imposed from above and not evolved by the farmers themselves. Simoons also criticizes Harris for ignoring or dismissing religiopolitical factors. For example, Harris claims that the concept of ahimsa has positive functions in that it confers material rewards; whereas Simoons points out that ahimsa operates in circumstances where there is no possibility of material reward.

The cultural ecologists press their case by referring to the importance of the cow in modern Indian economy. With deforestation in India dung has become an important source of fuel. Cow dung is a good fuel as it burns slowly and cleanly, and allows for food to be cooked while the family is in the fields. From 40% to 70% of all manure produced by Indian cattle is used as fuel for cooking. The rest is returned to the fields as fertilizer, forestalling the need for expensive chemical fertilizers. The energy equivalent of the dung used for cooking fuel is estimated at 43 million tons of coal and is an important saving on foreign exchange needed for other sources of fuel. More important even than this is the draught function. Oxen are still needed in huge numbers for farm work, and of course cows are needed to produce these work animals. During the dry season cows may become barren so the temptation to sacrifice them becomes greater. The prohibition against beef eating is thus a kind of insurance that farmers will not slaughter their cattle during this difficult time and that the agricultural system will recover when the rains come (Harris, 1974, 1978). Local governments maintain homes for barren cows; farmers reclaim, with a small fine, any cow that has calves or begins to lactate. Thus, the argument goes, ownership of cows is crucial to the well-being of rural peasants, for a farmer who loses a cow loses everything. Sharing of oxen is not practicable, because of seasonality and monsoons everyone needs them at the same time, and so every farmer ideally needs his own team. From this perspective there may be too few rather than too many cattle in India.

Although cows provide less than half the milk produced in India (most of them are not dairy breeds) their products, milk, curd, butter, dung and urine are regarded as having purifying properties. But despite its sacredness the cow is not treated particularly well by most Indians. Cows are left to scavenge while limited food will go to the oxen (though the cows will not be allowed to die). When they are sick they are worried over like sick children; decrepit beasts may just recover, while those that die from natural causes are in fact eaten by lower caste Hindus. The hide of the cow is also used in the extensive leather trade plied by the lower-caste Hindus. Even the bones may be processed for fertilizer. Given this economic usefulness, it may be thought that a better breed of cow could be introduced. Western agronomists claim that breeding programmes could produce stronger, healthier beasts capable of better work and of producing more milk. But the land that this would require is needed to produce food for people. In the US huge amounts of arable land are used to grow food for cattle and the energy inputs are enormous, whereas in India the cattle basically consume what is inedible for humans. By being allowed to wander freely, cows can scavenge, thus relieving the pressure on human food supplies. Also the Zebu cattle have adapted to their erratic climate; they can survive drought and are highly resistant to diseases. Like camels, they store water and food in their humps. An economic observer points out that 17% of the energy consumed by zebus is returned in the form of milk, traction and dung. American cattle raised on Western style ranges return only 4% (Odend'hal, 1972).

Cultural ecologists, then, view the cow complex as being the outcome of positive functioned adaptations to ecological and technological conditions rather than to the negative influence of religious concepts. It is a cultural mechanism to ensure that economic resources are protected.

Rejection of the social and religious aspects of cow keeping, however, weaken this thesis, for such functions have been amply demonstrated. The Sacred Cow taboo has developed from a complex history of religious thought, political exigencies and economic and environmental adaptations. It may be a mistake to try to separate these elements in attempts to justify an apparently irrational practice in rational terms. What is certain is that the persistence of the taboo over several hundreds of years indicates that it plays an important part in maintaining and portraying deeply held values in Indian society.

Cannibalism

Anthropophagy, or man-eating, is the term used by anthropologists to describe the eating of humans, or parts of them, by other humans. The term cannibalism is a corruption of carib, the name of an indigenous tribe encountered by Spanish colonialists in the 16th century. Columbus was informed by the Arawak Indians he landed among on his first voyage to the New World that their neighbours to the south, the Caribs, were an aggressive people who ate their prisoners. Columbus was not personally ready to believe these stories, noting that the Arawak also thought that he and his crew were cannibals. Nevertheless, despite the fact that he never witnessed the practice himself, his published accounts in Europe did pass on as fact the existence of cannibals in the New World. Brutish rumours steadily grew and were embellished by later explorers and missionaries. Hogg (1961) presents a survey of anecdotal evidence collected by early travellers, though for Arens (1979) that is the very problem; almost all the evidence for anthropophagy is second or third-hand. The ascription of cannibalism to others has always served to distinguish clear cultural boundaries, but there is no reliable first-hand evidence that it was ever a customary practice in any culture. Nevertheless, the halting of this 'barbarous practice' was often used as an excuse by would-be conquistadors to subdue native peoples.

Prevalent in many parts of Africa in the 1950s was the belief that white Europeans ate the flesh of Africans. This was bolstered by the appearance in the Belgian Congo of European canned meats with labels showing healthy African babies, and the introduction of cheap canned meat labelled 'For African Consumption' into Northern Rhodesia (Malawi). In the latter cases rumours suggested that the cans contained human flesh and were meant to break down local resistance to the idea of a Central African Federation. Lewis (1986) recounts that when a European commissioner publicly ate the canned meat to prove it was harmless it simply confirmed the African's suspicions that Europeans were cannibals.

Anthropologists have ascribed several possible functions to the practice of cannibalism. Religious, magical, and dietetic motivations are interwoven in the explanations offered, as is the quest for vengeance. The nutritional value of cannibalism is a favourite theory used to lend rational weight to the practice, the claim being made that it provided at least a partial answer to the problem of scarce animal protein supplies. However, although the possibility of ritual cannibalism may be admitted, it is unlikely that it could have ever been a significant source of nutrients. Lewis (1986) seeks to understand cannibalism as a symbolic practice which is an integral part of ritual life and dismisses materialist explanations based on protein deficiency. In a ritual setting, '... a tabooed negative action – eating human flesh – acquires positive force, the ritual consumption of the human body enables the consumer to acquire something of the body's vital energy'. Among several groups who allegedly practised cannibalism there was a belief that by swallowing the dead one could reabsorb the power or life essence that would otherwise be lost. A tribe could thereby retain the skills of members who had died or could take possession of an enemy's vitality.

Aren's trenchant criticism of the cannibal thesis throws doubt on the veracity of reported case studies of cannibalism. Rumours, fears, suspicions and accusations abound – but there is little solid ethnography. Anthropologists typically report that the people they lived among were cannibals 'long ago, before contact, until pacification, just recently or only yesterday' (Arens, 1979). Reports of cannibalism continue to serve the need to draw cultural boundaries, to distinguish between a civilized 'us' and a barbaric 'them'.

Modern anthropophagy

In recent history incidents of cannibalism have usually been connected with questions of survival. In conditions of severe hardship survival becomes an overall priority, and when the only hope of survival lies in anthropophagy the practice is generally sanctioned. The bitter retreat of Napoleon's army from Moscow; the famines which swept the Ukraine in the 1930s and 1940s; the Siege of Leningrad during the Second World War; all provide examples of humans overcoming their revulsions and breaking the taboo. In the late 19th century the pioneering Donner party, who were caught in a snow storm in the Sierra Nevada mountains, kept half their number alive to see California through the expediency of cannibalism.

A celebrated case in 1972 involved the crash of an aeroplane in the Andes, whereby members of the Uruguayan rugby team were stranded for over 10 weeks (Read, 1974). In subsequent public admissions that cannibalism was the means by which they had endured, the survivors claimed that their actions had been inspired by the fact that Jesus had shared His flesh and blood at the Last Supper and that eating of the dead had represented an intimate communion between them all. In the same year, 1972, a Canadian Arctic pilot, Martin Hartwell, ate the flesh of a dead nurse when his plane crashed in the wastes of the Northwest

Territories. In 1979, another plane accident led Brent Dyer and Donna Johnson of Saskatchewan, to eat parts of their dead father's body. In 1994, starving slum dwellers in Olinda, Brazil were reported to be eating human body parts found at a local garbage dump. Over a thousand poor families had built shacks on the dump and eked out a living by collecting and selling garbage, sometimes coming across bodies or body parts – which the mayor of Olinda described as either murdered people or medical refuse from hospitals.

What is possibly the most extensive episode of cannibalism in this century allegedly took place in the remote Guangxi province of China in the 1960s, though there has been no independent investigation to confirm documentary evidence. Red Guards and Communist officials are said to have tortured then ate victims labelled as counter-revolutionaries. School principals were killed, cooked and eaten by students; government-run cafeterias displayed bodies dangling on meat hooks and served human flesh to employees. At least 137 people, possibly hundreds more, were eaten, with the number of cannibals being in the thousands. The motivation seemed to be an ideological one of demonstrating revolutionary correctness.

SUMMARY

There is no society where people are permitted to eat everything, everywhere, with everyone and in all situations (Cohen, 1968). Prohibitions vary in cultural importance and hence in the vigour with which they are enforced. Persons breaking cultural taboos are liable to some sort of punishment ranging from disapproval, scorn, a fine, ostracism or prison, to death. The more severe sanctions are reserved for breaking of taboos involving flesh foods. Usually, compulsion is not necessary to maintain dietary taboos. 'Most individuals feel more secure when they are conforming to the standards of their own cultural system, which they view as being superior to all other...more rational, more logical, more practical, more noble.' (Cohen, 1968).

Sometimes the reasons why particular foods are circumscribed are obvious pragmatic ones related to questions of availability or of potential danger. In many cases though the rationale for food prohibitions, taboos and superstitions is far from clear and it is easy then to make the assumption that no good rationale ever existed. Historical analysis of taboos such as that of the Sacred Cow reveal the error of making these kind of assumptions. There is a tendency for us to want to explain every phenomenon in terms acceptable to objective science and because of this we often impose our own materialistic interpretations on cultural behaviours which defy our notions of commonsense. It is difficult of course, when looking in on a culture from the outside, to understand the practices of that culture, and so much more difficult to comprehend the value of those practices in the context of an earlier epoch. To compound the difficulty, we find that often earlier practices have been adopted and adapted by subsequent generations and invested with new meanings. If we look merely at the current manifestation of a given prohibition we see only a snapshot in time; taken out of the context of the entire album it is not surprising that that snapshot is incomplete and thus often misleading. Perhaps though, instead of trying to choose between religious or ecological, political, health or economic explanations for taboos and prohibitions we should recognize that each of these have had their part to play in the gradual evolution of the food practices we see today. Thus we can acknowledge that even seemingly irrational practices are cultural products, and that dietary change is inseparable from cultural change.

FURTHER READING

Simoons (1961) details the origin and diffusion of flesh avoidance in the Old and New Worlds.

For an example of the heated debate over the roles of material determinism and religion in the maintenance of the sacred cow taboo, see Freed, S.A. and Freed, R.S. (1981) Sacred Cows and Water Buffalo in India: The Uses of Ethnography, *Current Anthropology*, **22**(5): 483–90. The Freeds' article is followed by reactions from 18 anthropologists, supporting or critiquing (sometimes both) their work.

The role of the cow in contemporary Hindu rituals and popular sentiment surrounding the animal are described by Batra, S.M. (1986) The Sacredness of the Cow in India, *Social Compass*, **XXIII**(2–3): 163–75.

An account of the Peter Hartman story is given by Peter Tadman (1991), *The Survivor*, Gorman and Gorman, Hanna.

The story of Brent Dyer and Donna Johnson is told by Peter Gzowski (1980), *The Sacrament*, McClelland and Stewart Ltd., Toronto.

DISCUSSION QUESTIONS

1. Give examples of modern food myths or folklore in your own culture. What are the origins and impact of these myths?
2. Many food prohibitions and taboos apply only to women. Suggest reasons for this, providing some examples.
3. Discuss the materialist argument that the management of cattle in India represents a rational use of resources and therefore doesn't need religion to explain it.
4. Why is cannibalism 'good to think' despite the apparent lack of reliable evidence for its practice?

CHAPTER 9

Psychological aspects of food choice

We have already seen that people eat not only to meet physiological needs but also in response to social needs and pressures. To these we can now add a third dimension of psychological needs. Hunger and appetite are intimately connected to emotional needs. Emotional sensations such as yearning, craving, and compulsion give rise to patterns of eating behaviour which are gauged to relieve anxiety or tension, to provide security and comfort, or to provoke anger and frustration in others. Emotional responses to food develop early in childhood and are long-lasting; indeed, an infant's earliest pleasurable associations are with food; rooting and sucking reflexes which are associated with food-getting provide emotional contentment as well as physical nourishment. Feeding relieves unpleasant hunger pangs and produces feelings of well-being and satiety; thus babies quickly learn to equate eating with comfort. Food gratification is important in shaping an infant's future attitudes to food and sharing, and the foundations for healthy eating habits may be laid by provision of positive food experiences early in life.

Foods acquire particular associations through the circumstances in which they are commonly offered or eaten; for example, children quickly learn that sweetness equals love. When a new food is tasted it evokes an emotional response along the attraction/repulsion continuum which will influence its immediate and future acceptability. The nature of a foodstuff – its sweetness or bitterness for example – gives rise to physical sensations of pleasure or pain by direct sensory stimulation. Subsequent recall of these sensations also contributes to the ultimate labelling of a food as being pleasant or unpleasant. Such judgements regarding acceptability may be made merely from the look or smell of the food or even from pictures and photographs; actual consumption is not essential in order for pleasant or unpleasant associations to be made. Repeated experiences with a food fix its position in the constellation of feelings; thereafter, that food has the power to provoke emotional responses through the recall of particular or accumulated experiences of it.

Psychological states are frequently expressed through the use of food words. The primary tastes – sweet, bitter, sour and salty – are all used to describe personalities or temperaments; sweet has positive connotations while bitter and sour have definite negative connotations; salty is a less commonly used descriptor and its associations are not as obvious, though in some parts of Britain it denotes wit. Food features prominently in proverbs and sayings; a few common food metaphors and phrases are listed in Table 9.1.

Table 9.1 Food metaphors

Sweetheart
Sourpuss
Apple of my eye
Peaches and cream complexion
Bad egg
Cool as a cucumber
Cheesed off
Salt of the earth
Top banana
Big cheese
Brown as a berry
Breadwinner
Butter and eggs man
Butterfingers
Smart cookie
Like a fish out of water
As keen as mustard
Sweet as a nut
Mealy mouthed
Sugar daddy

FOOD AND EMOTIONS

There was once an advertisement on British TV which depicted a family at the breakfast table. Although everyone else was smiling and happy, the teenage daughter moodily pushed her bowl of cereal aside, untouched, while the voice-over pronounced: 'Susan? Well, Susan's in love.' This vignette of family life exemplifies the manipulation of emotional values of food in order to sell a product; happiness and laughter were associated with consumption of the product while a touch of humour was added by recognising the effect of lovesickness on teenage eating behaviour. It is perhaps useful to note that eating behaviour can be used actively, to express a particular feeling or state of mind, or passively as a reflection of an emotional state. In the first instance the behaviour is usually quite deliberate and its effect is calculated; in the latter case it is a subconscious response to internal needs.

Boredom

Eating may be used as a way to avoid or to stave off boredom. When there is nothing to do the refrigerator beckons and the larder stocks seem to take on a peculiar attraction. Food may be picked at or eaten in quantity, not because of hunger or appetite but simply for the sake of keeping occupied. Perhaps related to this is the idea of eating as a displacement activity. When studying gets just too tedious for words the answer is to make a cup of tea or a sandwich; when the lecturer drones on and on, or the car journey seems interminable, a packet of mints quickly disappears.

Loneliness

An emotionally insecure person may eat as a substitute activity for seeking love and affection. The idea that 'nobody loves me' leads naturally to the thought that 'it doesn't matter what I look like'. If nobody cares what does it matter if appearance suffers; hence whole cakes and chocolate bars are consumed yet hardly tasted. Repetitive behaviour of this kind triggers off feelings of guilt which in turn produces conditioned food responses. Eating can be a way to ward off depression, of cheering oneself up after a bad experience or a hard day. Often too, alcohol fulfils this function. Food and drink relieve frustration by substituting for desired love or affection. Older people may capture symbolically through food, the rewarding and nurturing experiences of earlier life.

Anxiety

Anxiety also leads to compensatory eating for comfort. Changed patterns of eating by students during exam week are related to anxiety and have both physical and emotional components. Butterfly stomachs leading to reduced appetite make large meals seem unappealing so that commonly, sweet high-calorie chocolate bars and soft drinks are substituted as they are more readily digestible. The emotional associations of these foods also connote comfort and reassurance. Adolescents often use food to restore emotional balance after a crisis; food provides transitory gratification until life settles down again. Chronic anxiety or depression may lead to obsession with a problem and food is then eaten compulsively. Whatever is chosen is defined as good because it leads to immediate gratification and the food retains this association even when the problem or crisis no longer exists. This type of behaviour can contribute to outcomes such as obesity.

An example from another culture, that of the Gurage people of Ethiopia, illustrates connections between food and anxiety. During early milk feeding and weaning Gurage children are exposed to a pattern of alternating glut and want; this, combined with the emotional detachment shown by parents toward their children, may explain the extreme anxiety exhibited by adults toward their food supply. Over-consumption and obesity among people living in a land of plenty have sometimes been ascribed to residual anxieties about hunger stemming from earlier experiences.

Guilt

The hardships of therapeutic diets may sometimes produce guilt reactions which are ultimately counter-productive. A large proportion of would-be slimmers cheat on their diets. Usually the cheating is clandestine and is not readily admitted to; the dieter continues to protest to not understanding why there is no weight loss and maintains that he or she is following the diet faithfully. Guilty feelings over such deception may lead to identification of the forbidden sweets and treats as good and desirable, and thereby their consumption is justified. In another type of therapeutic situation a mother may feel guilty at depriving her diet-bound child of a favourite food and in an effort to compensate puts the whole family on the diet.

Guilt feelings may be related to a failure to adhere to parental expectations. Immigrant Jewish mothers in New York in the 1930s implored their children to eat and become fat as they reasoned that fat children would not get tuberculosis. These children, as adults, then felt guilty if they did not overeat (Bruch, 1974).

Food is sometimes offered as a gift to assuage guilt. Thus a box of chocolates is offered to redress a wrongdoing; food parcels substitute for personal visits; ice-cream treats follow childhood chastisements. Is it possible to see in the fruit basket bought to the bedside of the sick an element of guilt, analogous to the guilt felt by survivors towards those who die?

Weapons and crutches

Food can be used as an emotional weapon by children, who quickly learn to wield the power gained from uncooperative eating behaviour. Not eating is a certain way of getting attention; by being overly fussy a child may learn to expect a reward as a bribe for desired behaviour. Food wars are a source of ill-feelings, anger and frustration. To the child they represent attempts to achieve control of the environment; the thwarting of the child's wishes confirms the dominance of adults and builds a sense of impotence and dependence. To the adult, the child's rejection of food symbolizes rejection of love and of parental authority. By not eating what he or she is told is good for them the child questions the adult's competency and knowledge of what is best. Adolescents too can show defiance and assert independence by rejecting previously accepted foods.

The emotional importance of food is well summarized in the following passage. 'Adults too frequently use food as an emotional outlet – a crutch to help them handle and to live with anxiety, tension, frustration, unhappiness, irritability, disappointment, loneliness or boredom. No human can escape such emotions as these and thus he must find ways to cope with them. Using food as a compensation mechanism to help one get rid of these emotions or accept their inevitability and learn to live with them may seem a bit ridiculous at first glance – but consider the alternatives. Few people are self-disciplined enough to make no alteration in their behaviour when under emotional stress except to keep an unusually stiff upper lip. Thus they resort to some kind of protective mechanism. They drink or take drugs; they whine or complain to elicit sympathy; they take it out on someone else by being cross or disagreeable; they wallow in self-pity. Compared to these destructive mechanisms, altering one's eating patterns would seem to be fairly innocuous.' (Gifft, Washbon and Harrison, 1972).

WEIGHT DISTURBANCES

The point made above is an interesting one to keep in mind when discussing the concept of poor eating habits. All too often only physical parameters and consequences are used to judge the value and desirability of eating habits. This is certainly almost always the case with the current medical opinion on being overweight. Although the considerable effort which is devoted to treatment and prevention of obesity is predicated largely on the desirability of preventing physical health problems it is at least partly a reflection of current norms of slimness in society. In other cultures, and at other times when obesity has been positively valued, such rigorous efforts have been absent. For many people who face the daily ordeal of diet and exercise, health is merely a by-product of a fashionable body image rather than an end in itself. Whatever the motivation though, the maintenance of a body weight which conforms to fairly narrowly defined limits is generally seen to be desirable. Inappropriate food choices may lead in the long term to physiological body states which are considered to be abnormal.

Obesity and anorexia nervosa are conditions which result from, or lead to, food consumption patterns which are divorced from actual physiological need. It is not within the scope of this book to discuss extensively either of these conditions but it is perhaps worth noting that psychological mechanisms, some of which have been already alluded to, play an integral part in the genesis or maintenance of abnormal body weight. The short discussion which follows identifies some common themes.

Obesity

The aetiology of obesity is complex and, despite extensive research studies and experimentation, is only poorly understood. Explanations range from the deterministic role of genetics, through social expectation theories, to psychological responses to personal needs. Deterministic theories which view obesity as being a product of genetic inheritance and biochemical make-up (e.g. the brown fat theory) tend to induce a fatalistic attitude whereby obese persons see themselves as the hapless, and helpless, victims of body chemistry. Such an outlook not only destroys feelings of personal control but also provides a ready-made excuse for failure in weight control efforts. At the other end of the spectrum, obesity is conceived of as a deliberately chosen condition to be used psychologically as a means of defence in a hostile world. Susie Orbach represents the latter view; claiming that fat is a feminist issue she interprets obesity in women as a kind of defence mechanism. Fat females are not pestered by men; they are not objects of aggressive sexual attention (Orbach, 1978). Other authors have commented that obesity can be used as a way to avoid the stresses of adult sexuality, particularly when it arises during the turbulent years of adolescence. Two distinct types of obesity, developmental and reactive, have psychological components. Developmental obesity stems from childhood and is associated with many other personality disturbances. Patients seen in obesity clinics, who have developmental origins to their obesity, are almost exclusively female and demonstrate high levels of anxiety, depression, social avoidance and somatic complaints as well as often declaring reduced interest in sexual activity. Reactive obesity occurs in more mature individuals as a response to some traumatic event in their lives, for example, a family bereavement.

Obesity can have important positive functions; for many people it is a compensatory mechanism in a frustrating and stressful life. Most commonly though, obesity is viewed negatively. There is no doubt that the cultural norm of slimness is so entrenched that for many deviation from this norm provokes feelings of guilt, unworthiness or rejection. Dissatisfaction with appearance, including body weight, is common especially among adolescents. Responses such as dieting, binging and purging (self-induced vomiting and use of laxatives and diuretics) seem to be occurring at younger and younger ages. Thousands of people devote substantial time, money and effort to achieve and maintain a socially acceptable weight. Their behaviour is reinforced by a medical establishment which emphasizes the negative health consequences of obesity and which chides overweight patients for lack of willpower and self-control. Paradoxically, in consumer societies, people receive a constant stream of messages telling them to eat; they are exhorted to consume but are punished for consuming.

The motivation necessary for an obese individual to successfully lose weight must be provided by internal rather than external stimuli. Relaxation of the cultural demand for slimness would allow individuals to determine if they truly wished to lose weight or if they were in fact more psychologically, and perhaps even physically, comfortable at a higher weight. It would also, by the way, largely wipe out an entire sector of commercial food marketing.

Anorexia nervosa

Anorexia nervosa is an extreme example of the potential effect of psychological disturbances on eating behaviour. Although it has long been known and there are a number of historical accounts of the condition, anorexia nervosa has been reported with greatly increased frequency over the past decade. This may reflect a real increase in incidence, which some would relate to the stressfulness of modern life, or it may be the result of more accurate diagnosis and better documentation and reporting procedures.

Although the results of anorexia nervosa are manifested as extreme inanition and emaciation, and are thus of vital concern to nutritionists, the aetiology of the disorder is rooted in psychological disturbances. Most common among adolescent females, primary anorexia nervosa is interpreted as a struggle for self-identity; non-eating and the subsequent drastic weight loss are late features of the disorder and are only secondary to underlying personality conflicts. Bruch (1974), in her seminal work on the subject, identified three areas of disturbed psychological functions. The first of these concerns delusions regarding body image. Some anorexics deny the abnormality of their emaciated state believing that their extreme thinness is desirable and normal, and they thus reject the need to eat. (This contrasts with a second group who recognize the undesirability of their physical condition but feel powerless to do anything about it.) Anorexics become very knowledgeable about the energy value of foods and are careful not to eat anything which might increase their weight. They resort to strategies such as lying, concealment of food, and self-induced vomiting to avoid food consumption and subsequent weight gain. The second disturbance is manifested as distorted perception or interpretation of internal body stimuli. Thus hunger pains are denied and there is a failure to recognize physiological need for food. Subsequently there are changes in food preferences, tastes, eating habits and manners; in addition, anorexics exhibit hyperactivity and denial of fatigue. Thirdly, there is an overwhelming sense of incompetence and ineffectiveness; anorexics perceive themselves as being reactive rather than proactive. While endeavouring to prevent continued weight loss, therapy is concerned mostly with achieving psychological stability.

Some common elements which emerge in case history studies of anorexics indicate that they often are well-educated and come from middle-class homes; as children they are responsible and dependable; parental expectations of them are high. Perfectionist attitudes and a desire to please are common, resulting in a subordination of self. Control is exercised by a dominant and over-protective mother, producing excessive dependency and unquestioning obedience. Anorexia nervosa may then be seen as an act of parental defiance; it is a way of asserting control over one's own body and thus over one's own life. Bruch gives central importance to this struggle for control. There is also a psychosexual element in the anorexic's behaviour which can be interpreted as a rejection of adult womanhood. Severe loss of weight results in amenorrhoea and retardation in development of secondary sex characteristics. By retaining a childlike figure the anorexic denies adult sexuality which is challenging and a threat to maintenance of self-control. As a disorder of gender identity, anorexia nervosa paradoxically combines both the search for an ideal body and the denial of womanhood.

As with obesity, anorexia nervosa cannot be approached as simply an eating disorder of individuals, but must be seen in a broader cultural context. Perimenis (1991) uses a content analysis of TV commercials to demonstrate stereotypical views of women as being preoccupied with body image. Anorexia is thus an expression of the social construction of gender.

A different perspective is introduced by scholars who locate anorexia nervosa within a female tradition of asceticism. Throughout history women have always undertaken dietary asceticism to construct an acceptable self. This was true in ancient Greece, among female religious groups in Medieval times and now among young women generally. Such behaviours may be part of the means by which age and sex differentiation is achieved. However, anorexia has been taken out of its religious context and bought into the medical realm, making it susceptible to the application of medical expertise and control. From a feminist perspective this might be another example of a dominantly male profession attempting to control women.

FOOD AND PSYCHOLOGICAL SECURITY

In examining Maslow's hierarchy of human needs it was earlier noted that food security followed basic survival as the next rung on the upward ladder of need–achievement. Security implies a lack of anxiety over where the next meal is coming from. Emotional growth in infancy is nurtured by undisrupted routines, thus regular meals are necessary for a happy child. Early lack of security may give rise to fussiness and eating difficulties in later life. Food is one of the major gratifications one receives on entering the world. It relieves bodily discomfort and provides comforting body contact. A mother's treatment of the feeding process, be it relaxed, fidgety or fearful will determine the infant's first impressions of the world.

In times of crisis, familiar foods are highly valued. Certain foods commonly represent comfort and security. Milk, being the universal first food of humans, often takes on this role and people have strong emotional attitudes to milk. Harriet Bruce Moore (1952) spoke of: 'the unhappy, suffering, far from home and loved ones, soldier [who] looks back to milk as in many ways expressing the comfort security and contentedness of life as it was at home'. For other groups different foods symbolize this security. In the last century early missionaries to Hawaii waited impatiently for sailing vessels to arrive from their native Massachusetts, bringing more supplies of their familiar wheat flour and salt pork. After a 6-month trip around the Horn the flour was often weevily and the pork rancid; but it was consumed with relish whereas the diet of Taro, fresh fruit and fish eaten by native Hawaiians was rejected (Gifft, Washbon and Harrison, 1972). Familiarity often makes a food more acceptable and sought after. Perhaps historically, familiarity served as a protective device to guard against poisoning with unfamiliar substances, though, as we shall see, variety in the diet could only be obtained by experimenting with unfamiliar foods. Young children much prefer familiar foods when they are in strange surroundings. Immigrants use familiar foods as a means of feeling secure and not losing their identity in a foreign land, and are often willing to pay high prices for these familiar symbols of home.

Hoarding

After survival needs have been met, ensuring security of food supply is an important human activity. Hoarding behaviour is a reflection of anxiety about security of the future food supply. Shack (1971), in his account of the Gurage of Ethiopa, refers to their hoarding of the food crop, ensete, during times of plenty. This, he suggests, is in response to their memories of fear during times of shortage and is a reflection of food insecurity. Similar hoarding behaviour has been observed in other societies which have a glut and famine existence. Food is stored against potential disaster and to this extent it is an adaptive behaviour, though when carried to excess it has negative repercussions.

The typically excessive storage of food by modern Europeans and Americans, which is usually done for overt reasons of cost-effectiveness and convenience, may contain an element of security–anxiety. Certainly when food shortages threaten people are easily panicked into buying and hoarding commodities. For example, a sugar shortage in Britain in the 1970s resulted in thousands of perfectly normal and reasonable people fighting openly in supermarkets to obtain the limited supplies available. Staff were abused for rationing what was available, and generally customers acted with complete lack of consideration for the needs of others. This kind of reaction to shortages may occur even when the shortage is imaginary or overplayed by reporting in the mass media. Film footage in news reports provides visible evidence that a product is not readily available and thus increases the panic demand even further. It is not unknown for food corporations to withhold supplies for short periods in an attempt to deliberately induce panic buying. Certainly, it is common practice for powerful corporations to withhold staple commodities from the market until the price is judged to be right.

Over-feeding of children may be in some instances a security response by parents who have themselves experienced food shortages. They are determined that their children will not suffer the same privations. The concept of obesity as a form of personal hoarding may sound strange but we know that over-eating is often linked to feelings of unhappiness and anxiety, and is a source of comfort and solace. Cohen (1961) comments that in a society where the young are not fed on demand, adults will tend to hoard food and wealth. Early food gratification creates an emotional predisposition to share food. Food symbolizes social interactions and serves to meet the psychological need for interchange. Weinberg (1972) sees hoarding by the elderly as an attempt to hold onto to things previously shared in intimacy with others, through the symbolism of food.

Stress and food selection

Animals under conditions of stress may substitute one instinctual behaviour for another. Similarly, it is possible that humans utilize eating as an alternative response to 'fight or flight' when threatened.

Dieting may itself be a source of stress. Attempts to maintain a lower body weight and the constant worry over gaining a pound or two results in anxiety and tension and a lessened ability to cope emotionally. Increased irritability as a side effect of dieting is familiar to all those who have suffered the martyrdom of family or friends who decide to slim down. Any change in eating patterns, in that it upsets familiar practices, produces at least some emotional tension. Where the change is imposed or made in response to external motivators the resulting stress will be greater than when changes are made deliberately to meet personal goals.

Personality and food choice

The stereotype of the fat jolly person is a persistent one, and it lends popular credence to the idea that personality is somehow related to food consumption. If one were to investigate the basis for the stereotype it might be found that fat people assume jolliness as a defence or as a social integration mechanization; or it may be that people who are jolly indulge in more social eating events and therefore tend to become fat; or it may be that there is really no basis for the stereotype at all. The effect of personality on food behaviour, or vice versa, has not been well studied. Murray and Watson (1978) used the Eysenck Personality Inventory to investigate food preferences of introverts and extroverts. They found that introverts had significantly more food dislikes than did extroverts. There was no relationship found between neuroticism and food dislikes, though other studies have reported an association of neuroticism with thinness.

Thinness has also been associated with schizophrenia, sadness and tension states. Whereas fatness may be linked to lower levels of anxiety and depression, there is little evidence of clear relationships between obesity and psychiatric status.

Food may be used as a way of demonstrating mood either through the care taken over food preparation or by the refusal to eat food prepared by others. The latter behaviour is an obvious sign of anger or annoyance. Older children will sometimes refuse previously liked foods as a means of regaining the attention they feel has been usurped by the arrival of a younger sibling. In adolescence and in adulthood food choice can be a reflection of self-image; conformity or individualism can be displayed through eating behaviour. As previously noted, the consumption of health foods or the practice of vegetarianism may be expressions of certain values regarding the world. Because the reaction to the hunger drive is so visible in its effects it is not surprising that it has social significance in assignment of identity to an individual. Advertisers play on this social need by encouraging identification with a product or particular brand. What you buy and what you eat tells others that you are discerning, thrifty or extravagant, modern or old-fashioned. In this way food choice becomes a manifestation of personality.

FOOD PREFERENCES

Food preferences function as a means of assessing the acceptability of foods, preference implying a degree of like or dislike. Preference also implies an expressed choice rather than merely a willingness to eat a food and preferences may indeed differ from actual consumption patterns. Foods may be accepted even though they are not preferred, for reasons of availability, cost or social courtesy. When our favourite fruit, fresh strawberries, is out of season, we buy frozen ones or choose different fruits; when prime cuts of meat cost more than the wallet can bear we settle for chops or stew; when our new-found friends invite us to dinner and serve up lasagna, we don't admit that we loathe pasta, but take the smallest portion and comment on how nice it is (at the same time politely but firmly declining second helpings). The rarity with which people bother to enquire about specific food dislikes of others suggests that either they see their own tastes as reflecting majority tastes or that they are more concerned with what the dish says about themselves than with their guest's pleasure. (On numerous occasions I have been expected to enjoy elaborate meat dishes when no-one had the foresight to ascertain that I was a vegetarian.)

It is sometimes argued that the body knows what is good for it and that given a free choice humans would automatically select nutritionally adequate diets. To test this idea in conditions where cultural learning was minimal, Davis (1928,1939) experimented with allowing newly weaned infants to choose their own diets from a selection of offered foods. She found that definite preferences were shown which changed unpredictably from time to time; appetite was the guiding factor and the diets consumed were nutritionally adequate, but probably only because the selection of nutritious foods offered made it difficult for this not to happen. A recent re-evaluation of Davis's studies is provided by Story and Brown (1987). There are of course ethical problems with this type of study but it is unlikely that, given a completely free choice of foods, an infant would select a nutritionally adequate diet. Young children do adjust their food choices when they are conscious of parental monitoring, at least to reduce foods which they believe are not approved of (Klesges *et al.*, 1991).

Food preferences are shaped in early life by culturally determined patterns in which foods are consumed in specific combinations and which reflect experiences and associations made largely within the sphere of influence of the family. However, parent–child resemblance in preferences appears, paradoxically, to be low. If children learn their food preferences from their culture one might expect the parental influence to be greater; if within-culture variance is environmental but not familial, then where does it come from? (Rozin, 1990). Simple exposure to foods is a key element in their acceptance. All foods are initially unfamiliar to a child, who must learn what they taste like and that they are safe to eat. Birch (1992) suggests that a minimum of eight to ten exposures is necessary before a child accepts a food. Actual ingestion is necessary so that the child learns that there are no negative physiological consequences. This calls for persistence on the part of parents in offering new foods.

Children seem to prefer high-fat foods, which are both widely availability and culturally valued. In the US, Agras *et al.* (1988) reported that children as young as 18 months preferred foods, such as hot dogs, with high quantities of fat and salt. High-fat foods are ubiquitous as snacks and as fast food and are provided in positive social circumstances. Children may be attracted to the sweet taste of the sugar often found in combination with, and masking the taste of, fats and find the actual foods pleasant and satiety-inducing. If children are exposed predominantly to high-fat foods then this is what they will learn to like.

Pilgrim (1957) carried out extensive studies on food preferences of men in the US armed forces. Among other things he was interested in the practical question of whether or not food preferences could be used to predict actual food consumption and thus help to reduce food wastage. Despite the reservations noted earlier, preference and actual choice do seem to be positively related; where food choice is not limited by income it seems logical to assume that people will choose the foods they prefer. Preference and actual food consumption become more congruent with increasing affluence. Food preferences are affected by three sets of factors;

those associated with the food itself, with the individual eater, and with the environment. While these must certainly be to some extent interactive they are for convenience of discussion treated separately below.

Characteristics of the food

The sensory qualities of food are important in determining what is preferred, though highly preferred foods will sometimes be avoided if there is an unpleasant visceral experience associated with their consumption. Thus it is not uncommon to hear someone say something along the lines of: 'Oh yes, I like it – but it doesn't like me'. The organoleptic or inherent sensory properties of a food such as its visual appearance, smell, taste and texture shape individual preferences, as do the way in which the food is prepared and its ease of eating.

For example, appropriate colour is used as an index of normality, of maturity, of purity and of quality. Colour also influences perception of sweetness and thus of acceptability. Texture, flavour and odour are other indexes of appropriateness, of deterioration and of proper cooking technique as illustrated in Table 9.2. Most people have a mental construct of what constitutes perfection in any given food or dish; when offered these foods they match them against the ideal in order to determine their acceptability. Thus a food may be quite edible, but, because it falls short of perfection it is rejected and labelled as undesirable and unfit. Children commonly refuse to eat even preferred foods because they don't 'look right', or because they are 'not cooked properly'. Ironically, we often accept lower standards of perfection when we are paying more for food, as is the case in restaurants. Perhaps cognitive dissonance dictates that in order to justify high expenditures on a restaurant meal we have to convince ourselves mentally that the food was really worth it, whatever our taste buds tell us. Or perhaps we just lower our expectations. Fortunately, children usually do not make such compromises and reject unsatisfactory dishes whether eating at home, Aunty Mary's, or the poshest restaurant in town.

Table 9.2 Organoleptic properties influencing preference for apples

	Colour	Flavour/odour	Texture
Appropriate	Red	Sweet	Crisp
Non-appropriate	Yellow	Sour	Soft
Deteriorated	Brown	Sour	Mushy
Fresh	Green	Sweet	Firm
Cooked properly	Clear	Sweet	Soft
Improperly cooked	Brown	Burnt	Bitty

Sensory evaluation of foods has become a huge area of interest for researchers and food manufacturers, much effort and money being expended on taste testing with consumer panels. Whatever the organoleptic merits of a single foodstuff, it is true that most foods are eaten in combination. The aesthetic qualities of meal composition have an effect on acceptability and degree of preference (Table 9.3). Similar aesthetic criteria may be applied to the judgement of a complete meal. Highly preferred foods may be avoided if served with inappropriate or unexpected accompaniments; hence the importance of pleasing menu combinations.

Table 9.3 Sensory attributes of a high quality mixed dish

Topography	Some large and small pieces so that when it is served it forms a pile.
Neatness	Pieces are cut uniformly and any sauce is not runny; no part extends beyond the edge of the dish.
Quantity	Reasonable in proportion to the dish – neither skimpy nor too much.
Harmony	A pleasing integration and arrangement of items; colours, textures, shapes, flavours, and odours are compatible.
Emphasis	Pleasing contrasts of colour, shape, texture, flavour and odour.

Based on information in Eckstein, E.F. (1980) *Food, People and Nutrition*, AVI, Westport.

Characteristics of the individual

Food dislikes are common in young children; taste sensitivity decreases in later years as numbers of taste buds decline, and this may have the effect of enhancing the acceptability of foods. Korslund and Eppright (1967) discovered that children with the lowest taste sensitivities tended to accept more foods, though evidence that taste acuity and preference are strongly related is lacking. There appears to be some sex difference regarding food preferences; for example, women have a greater preference for sour tastes, but it is not certain if apparent differences are real or culturally induced. It also seems that women have more food aversions than do men. Using hedonic scales of like–dislike, Pilgrim (1961) found that people tended to like or dislike groups of foods. Individuals of similar background gave similar responses. Age influenced food–class preference, though educational level was less important.

Characteristics of the environment

Although it is well recognized that environmental factors play a large part in determining food availability and indirectly therefore, choice, possible direct effects on food preference have not been extensively studied. Seasonality, urbanization and geographical area of origin and habitation may exert measurable effects, as do situational factors such as immediate physical surroundings. Food retailers and restaurateurs have long recognized the importance of physical surroundings and ambience in providing customers with pleasant and appropriate eating experiences. Thus fast-food chains often employ bright bold colours to signal their up-tempo brashness, whereas cosy candle-lit restaurants make the most of dark warm colours which invite the customer to linger.

It seems then, that those individualistic likes and dislikes which we collectively call food preferences are a product of cultural and biological factors. The question is still open as to whether we seek preferred foods or learn to like those foods which are available, though it would appear sensible to look for a way of reconciling the two. To this end the next section is devoted to a discussion of the interplay of culture and biology.

BIOLOGY AND CULTURE IN TASTE DEVELOPMENT

As tastes and acceptable food combinations are learnt early it is not surprising that in later life familiarity is an important factor in influencing preferences. However, humans also desire variety in the diet and thus new foods must be sampled – with the possibility that they will be unacceptable, repulsive or even dangerous. Competing desires for familiarity and novelty must somehow be reconciled. In different parts of the world there are characteristic flavour principles which are repetitively used in all basic food dishes: e.g. curry, chili, oregano. Rozin (1978) suggests that these flavours may be used to provide a familiar and reassuring flavour and thus blunt fear of the unknown while at the same time promoting acceptance of new foods. Variety is increased because within the overall flavour scheme there are many graduations of taste, just as there are considerable differences in the class of beverages known as wine. Repeated experiences with wine consumption lead to greater discrimination and changes in palatability; a wine which is initially rejected as being too dry may eventually become more acceptable than previously preferred sweet wines. Similarly, Europeans who learn to like curries may graduate from mild dishes to searingly hot ones as they become accustomed to the spicy taste sensations.

As omnivores seeking to maximize food availability, humans have relatively few genetic controls on food selection (Rozin, 1990), though genetic factors may lead to cultural learning of specific food preferences or avoidances. For example, genetically endowed enzyme deficiencies may lead to the avoidance of milk products and fava beans. There are however, some biological biases. Immediately after birth the human infant already prefers sweet tastes and has aversions to bitter and sour solutions; this preference for sweet flavours continues through adult life. The sweetness preference may be an adaptive behaviour for humans in their search for energy sources in the food environment; sweetness is associated with calories and thus with survival. The role of culture is to increase availability of, and amplify the basic biological preference for, sweetness. However, the adaptive liking for sweets in nature readily becomes a maladaptive over-reliance on sweets in modern urban societies, where availability overwhelms need.

In nearly every culture there is at least one innately unpalatable substance which becomes an important food or drink. Several authors have commented on the widespread use of chilli pepper as a condiment and on the use of coffee, which is universally served in North America for adults but which is disliked by children, who must be taught to like it. Unpalatability is often associated with plants which contain toxins and which therefore could be dangerous; a bitter taste may be a warning not to eat the plant. Most animals do avoid bitter or irritant foods and only humans persist in the use of a substance which they find distasteful on the first few encounters. This suggests that human reactions are culturally influenced. Chilli pepper is an innately unpleasant substance which has become very widely consumed; Rozin suggests that people do not eat chilli for any ulterior motive or benefit but do actually come to like the burning sensation it imparts. Initial forced exposure to chilli is followed by social reinforcement, which, combined with flavour enhancement gives rise to a real preference. He also speculates on the operation of an emotional homoeostasis system; the unpleasant taste of chilli is countered by an opposing effect reaction which gives rise to a pleasant internal sensation. With repeated exposures, this pleasurable opponent becomes dominant and thus chilli becomes liked. An explanation which invokes beneficial health effects as a rationale for consumption is offered by Pangborn (1975) who speculates that the widespread use of hot spicy foods is related to their bacteriostatic properties.

FOOD AVERSIONS AND CRAVINGS

The opposite side of the coin to food preference is food aversion. A term which implies something stronger than mere avoidance, aversion suggests an active distaste. This may begin merely as a food avoidance resulting from religious or social regulations, or simply as a personal dislike. A shared dislike for a food may turn it into something at first undesirable, then repellant, then detestable. Such is the case with insects and rodents as far as most Europeans and North Americans are concerned, though these same creatures are important food sources in Africa and other parts of the world (cf. Chapters 2 and 8). Potential food substances are primarily rejected because of disliked sensory characteristics (distaste), anticipated negative consequences (danger), offensive connotations (disgust) or classification of the substance as not edible.

Garb and Stunkard (1974) reported that the majority of people learn food aversions through the unpleasant physical experience of illness, usually gastrointestinal in nature. If stomach-upsets follow chronologically the consumption of a particular food, an association between the two events is readily made which may lead to permanent abstention from the food item concerned. Strong aversions may be formed to foods which have not even been tasted, as in the above examples of insects and rodents. Even a generous chocolate coating was not sufficient to induce students in one of my classes to try grasshoppers, while in another food class samples of squid were resolutely avoided in favour of familiar white fish. The idea of eating horsemeat and dogflesh provoke similar feelings of disgust in many people and yet they are perfectly acceptable foodstuffs to others. Patently, our ethnocentric views on what is food are culturally rather than biologically conditioned.

Food aversions are most common in children, being acquired between the ages of 6 and 12 years and declining in older age groups. Sometimes children's food avoidances are blamed on the mother for eating too much of the food during pregnancy. If there is any truth in this assertion it is probably because the food in question is not offered frequently at family mealtimes or because the mother attaches negative connotations to its consumption by recalling that she ate it until she was sick of it. Transient aversions, lasting only a few weeks, are also often seen among cancer patients receiving radiation therapy.

Substances normally judged to be inappropriate as food may be consumed under specialized circumstances. Wallpaper paste was eaten by the desperately hungry victims of the Siege of Leningrad; dandelion or marigold leaves may be used in salads, for effect or to demonstrate bush living. Cannibalism may be the only resort of those isolated through natural or man-made catastrophe. Inappropriateness is a cultural judgement which may be set aside if necessity dictates, as in survival situations, or to avoid giving offence when dining with hosts from a different culture.

Just as simple food dislikes may develop into disgust aversions so in some circumstances can food preferences be elevated to the rank of intense longings, or cravings. Cravings are often associated with the physiological status of pregnancy. Dickens and Trethowan (1971) studied cravings and aversions in a group of pregnant young English women; aversions identified most frequently were to tea, coffee, cocoa, vegetables, meat, fish and eggs. Cravings were strongest for fruit, fruit drinks, sweets, ice-cream, milk and dairy products. The authors comment that these desires were more common in women who were orally fixated. Hook (1978) also found that sweets, ice-cream, milk and fruit were frequently craved during pregnancy and that meats and poultry were more frequently avoided than craved. Both authors suggest that cravings and aversions of pregnancy may be due to changes in taste thresholds and sensitivity of smell. A more recent study of pregnant adolescents in the Southern US revealed similar patterns of cravings and aversions. Cravings were reported for sweets, especially chocolate, fruits and fruit juices, as well as for fast foods, pickles and ice-cream. The most common aversions were to meat, eggs and pizza (Pope, Skinner and Carruth, 1992).

The Doctrine of Maternal Impression held that any strong emotional state of the mother would be imprinted on the child. Wet nurses in Victorian England were screened for temper, sobriety and morality in the belief that temperament and passion could be passed through the milk during breastfeeding, thus rendering the child vulnerable to immoral habits. Similarly, connections are readily made between a mother's eating behaviour and real or supposed effects on the baby. Snow and Johnson (1978) studied a clinic population in Michigan and found a number of widespread folk beliefs concerning diet in pregnancy. Over two-thirds of the women in the study sample believed in the possibility of 'marking the child': a third of these respondents specifically mentioned food cravings as the source of the mark. For example, cherries or strawberries eaten by the pregnant woman could produce red spots on the infant. Most women gave examples in which unsatisfied cravings resulted in marking; for example, a woman with a craving for strawberries, who touched her cheek, would thereby cause a strawberry birthmark on the cheek of her infant. The authors offer a rationalization for this belief which says, in effect, that because birthmarks are out of the ordinary they must be explained; food cravings are associated with pregnancy in which the obvious physiological difference from the non-pregnant, non-craving state, is the presence of the foetus. Therefore it is easy to make the connection that it is the foetus which 'needs' the desired food, and which is then marked if its needs are unmet. Another example from Snow and Johnson's study was the reported belief that if a woman did not satisfy a craving for chicken then her baby would look like a chicken.

Pica

Pica is derived from the Latin word for magpie, a bird which eats anything, and is used to denote compulsive eating, particularly of substances which are non-nutritive such as dirt and clay. The term geophagy, meaning dirt-eating, is also used. Pica is commonly seen in the form of unusual cravings during pregnancy though it is by no means restricted to this physiological state. Hochstein (1968) identified six hypotheses to account for the practice of pica by pregnant women:

- **Psychological**: to get attention
- **Anthropological**: traditional behaviour taught by mothers to daughters during process of gardening and food preparation, which were women's tasks
- **Sensory**: clay eating decreases uterus movements and intestinal mobility and thus reduces nausea. It also reduces hunger
- **Microbial**: pica influences acidity of intestinal tract, favouring growth of normal organisms and discouraging that of pathogens
- **Physiological**: reduces amount of saliva in mouth which is a problem for some pregnant women
- **Nutritional need**: pica provides some nutrient missing from the diet

The evidence to give widespread support to any of these hypotheses is scanty. Various studies have indicated that pica is a culturally determined behaviour but there is disagreement as to its possible nutritional value. Fifty years ago Dickins and Ford (1942) reported that clay eating was common among Mississippi Negro schoolchildren and was viewed by them as a cultural practice. Vermeer and Frate (1975) say that the tradition of clay eating was so engrained in African ancestors of Southern US Negroes that its continuation was necessary for psychological well-being. Hunter (1973) also suggests that the practice was transplanted, via the slave trade, to the United States where cultural substitutes for the clay were found. Laundry starch, baking soda, wheat flour and dried powdered milks may be used as replacements. Clay eating is also seen as a cultural means of symbolically strengthening well-being among northern Australian aboriginal women who have made the transition from a nomadic to a settled lifestyle (Eastwell, 1979).

Several authors have postulated that clay eating has possible nutritional and medicinal benefits. Hunter (1973) suggests that minerals in clays eaten in Ghana act as dietary supplements, although Vermeer (1971) reported only small amounts of calcium in analysed clay samples from the same area. In contrast, this same researcher found considerable amounts of calcium and magnesium in clays eaten by pregnant Tiv women in Nigeria (Vermeer, 1966). Pica has been claimed to be both a cause and consequence of anaemia. Some clays may impair iron absorption (as well as that of potassium and zinc) and thus contribute to the development of anaemia, though there is little evidence that anaemia itself triggers geophagia. Solien (1954), like others, rejects the idea that dirt eating results from the body's recognition of a physiologic need for certain nutrients. Instead an ecocultural explanation is offered; dirt, which was used to quiet hunger pains during times of famine, became an acquired taste and so the practice was continued even when food became plentiful. It is also possible that earth was seen as a source of life and power and that magical thinking was involved in the deliberate consumption of part of that earth.

Many studies of pica have focused on low-income Blacks and indeed it is among this group that pica appears to be most prevalent. However, the practice has also been noted among low-income Whites, though higher socioeconomic groups have not been extensively studied. Explanations given by practitioners of pica for their behaviour include relief of nausea, social approval, tradition and expected physical effects on the baby. In Snow and Johnson's study some women thought that craving starch and clay indicated a dietary need but thought that taking too much would cause the child to be born covered with the excess as a caul. Finally, the idea that pica is an attention-getting stratagem is undermined by the finding that many women are reluctant and embarrassed to admit to the practice.

SUMMARY

Because eating is so often a social activity involving interaction with others it provides an ideal way in which to demonstrate mood and reflect emotions. Without having to say anything we can show that we are angry, bored, or anxious; we can demonstrate love and caring, disinterest or neglect. Eating behaviour is a form of non-verbal communication containing coded messages of great complexity and subtlety. The child's sudden refusal to eat says 'Give me some attention'; the anorexic teenager proclaims 'You cannot control me'; the obese young woman says (perhaps) 'Keep away!'. The same gesture might mean quite different things according to circumstance; for example, the gift of a box of chocolates could mean: 'I love you', 'I'm sorry', or 'I'm feeling guilty for neglecting you'. Caution is the watchword when attempting to interpret the language of food!

Psychological disturbances may sometimes be physically manifested as loss of weight control. Although it would be absurd to claim that all overweight people had other problems in coping with life, the possibility of psychological elements in the genesis of obesity should not be overlooked in the professional counselling and treatment of overweight patients. It is much more clear though, that the nutritional consequences of anorexia nervosa are symptomatic of underlying psychological disorders. While dietary treatment alone may be effective in treating obesity (though it rarely is) it is certainly not an adequate response to the serious condition of anorexia nervosa. Here we have a pre-eminent example of psychological stress producing changes in food choice behaviour, which in turn affect nutritional status and physical well-being.

Even in the absence of pronounced psychological aberrations food selection is a function of the way we think. Far from it being a rational activity designed to provide nutritional satisfaction in as efficient a manner as possible, choosing what to eat is a complex process governed to a great extent by mental deliberations; for there is ample evidence to show that we eat with our eyes and minds as much as with our taste buds and stomachs. There is some basis for claiming the existence of an inherent liking or dislike for certain tastes and flavour principles; sweetness is generally liked and desired, while bitterness is not. However, it is obvious that tastes can be acquired and thus that likes and dislikes are products of cultural learning. As they are learned, they confer acceptability on regularly consumed foods which leads to long-term preferences for familiar items. Thus even at the level of individual food selection it is difficult to maintain the illusion that objective free choice is likely. Of course it is possible to argue that we could choose to eat earthworms or goldfish if we really wanted to, but the very fact that we don't so choose seems to indicate that there are indeed restraints operating. My contention, repeated throughout this book, is that we understand very clearly that edible substances may be culturally classified as either food or non-food and we are careful to preserve this distinction in our personal eating habits.

FURTHER READING

For examples of commercially motivated scarcity, see Susan George (1976) *How the Other Half Dies*, Penguin Books, Middlesex, particularly the section entitled 'Planned Scarcity'. Also, Don Mitchell (1975) *The Politics of Food*, James Lorimer & Co., Toronto, provides examples of the manipulation of food supply and prices in a Canadian context.

Marilyn Lawrence (1987) *Fed Up and Hungry*, The Women's Press, London, presents a collection of essays on the relationship of women to food, including insights into eating disorders based on the work and personal experiences of the contributors.

For a Japanese perspective, see Baba, K. *et al.* (1985) Eating disorders in adolescence. *Jpn. J. Child. Adol. Psychiatr.*, 26(2): 86–115.

For discussion of anorexia from a perspective of ascetism and religion, see Tait, G. (1993) 'Anorexia Nervosa': Ascetism, Differentiation, Government. *Aust N.Z. J. Sociol.*, 29(2): 194–208.

Recent reviews of pica are provided by Lacey, E.P. (1990) Broadening the perspective of pica: literature review. *Public Health Rep.*, 105(1): 29–35; and by Horner, R.D., Lackey, C.J. Kolassa, K. and Warren, K. (1991) Pica practices of pregnant women. *J. Am. Diet. Assoc.*, 91(1): 34–8. The latter paper reviews 40 years of evidence for pica in pregnancy and demonstrates that it is still more prevalent than commonly believed. See also, Reid, R.M. (1992) Cultural and medical perspectives on geophagia. *Med. Anthropol.*, 13(4): 337–51.

Issues of taste development and genetics are explored in Barker, L. (ed.) (1982) *The Psychobiology of Human Food Selection*, AVI, Westport; and

Weiffenbach, J.M. (ed.) (1977) *Taste and Development. The Genesis of Sweet Preference Humans: Infants, Children and Adults,* Fogarty International Center Proceedings, No.32, NIH, Bethesda.

DISCUSSION QUESTIONS

1. Sometimes it is said that the body 'knows' what it needs. What is the evidence for specific nutrient hungers among humans?
2. Drawing from your own experience, discuss the notion of 'comfort foods'.
3. What role does parental influence play in the formation of food preferences, and what factors might affect the degree of this influence?
4. For most of human existence people have devoted much of their time to obtaining sufficient food to subsist; in contemporary Western societies they spend much of their time avoiding food. Discuss this in particular relationship to women and dieting.
5. Find evidence for, or speculate on, the effect of blindness on food preferences.

CHAPTER 10

Food for the masses

This chapter examines three situations where food is provided within large-scale enterprises. The first section is devoted to fast food, and in particular to what might be called the burger culture of North America. Fast food, despite its advertised quantity, is almost minimalist in nature; everything is reduced to its sparest, most utilitarian form. Social, psychological, even ideological meanings are still to be found but they are transformed by the rationalising process in which they are embedded. The second section describes a Japanese food phenomenon known as Ekiben, to illustrate how aesthetic and cultural food values can be preserved in the realm of mass feeding. The final section explores the world of airline food, demonstrating how the social status function of food is reproduced and to a large extent exacerbated in flight.

FAST FOOD – THE BURGER CULTURE

The growth of the fast-food industry, especially in North America, over the past 30 years has had a major effect on cultural foodways. Its impact can be measured primarily by the extent to which people eat away from the home, and the dominance of fast-food restaurants in this 'eating out' market. Fast foods generally refer to the products of fast-food restaurants, although 'restaurant' is perhaps a little misleading. Burgers and french fries, hot-dogs, fried chicken pieces, fish sandwiches, doughnuts, milk shakes and ice-cream are the cornerstones of fast food, albeit with a hundred slight variations.

The role of technological change

The emergence of fast-food restaurants as ubiquitous symbols of modern industrialized society has occurred in parallel with and, to a certain extent has been made possible by, rapid technological changes. Foremost among a bewildering array of such changes was the arrival of the car as an affordable family good, and its consequent dominance as an important, if not essential, family possession. With ready access to transport it becomes relatively easy to go out for a meal and, with a fast-food restaurant within a 3-minute drive for 50% of the American population, the choice of where to go is easy. To further cater to our mechanized habits (as well as to increase the profitability of the operation) many fast-food restaurants now provide a drive-through service.

There have been numerous advances in food technology which have revolutionized the nature of the food supply and which have had direct or indirect effects on food habits. Some of these changes made the idea of a fast-food restaurant first viable then increasingly profitable; others were developed especially to meet fast food needs. Preservation techniques such as drying and freezing, cooking methods such as microwaving, kitchen equipment for precise chopping, dicing and shaping of raw ingredients, equipment which monitors and controls temperatures, cooking times and 'doneness', machines which measure and deliver precise quantities – all have contributed to the revolution. To a large extent the modern fast-food restaurant resembles nothing so much as a heavily mechanized factory. These same technologies are now having an equally far-reaching impact on food preparation and eating habits in the home.

The market demand for vast quantities of standardized products has given rise to changes in the way food is grown and distributed. The huge purchasing power of fast-food restaurant chains allows them to dictate what is grown, where, of what quality and in what quantities. For example, a commercially preferred variety of potato is grown to the exclusion of traditional local varieties; beef cattle are raised in conditions such to ensure they have exactly the right type of meat; feed input, light and exercise conditions are closely controlled to ensure a consistent final product. In this way, fast-food chains achieve vertical integration, coming to control large chunks of the food supply system from production, through transportation to preservation, preparation, to consumption.

The advent of sophisticated computer technology has also contributed to the operation of fast-food restaurants. Computers can control cooking operations to an almost infinite degree, eliminating human error and deviations from absolute consistency. Pre-programmed computerized cash registers make it quick and easy for till clerks to enter orders, calculate costs and give change. Computers installed in drive-through counters now allow customers to punch in their own orders reducing waiting times and staffing overheads.

Scale of enterprise

Fast food and fast-food restaurants are congruent with and reflect prominent social values of speed, efficiency and conformity. They are seen to be cheap, clean and fun and they have come to symbolize the modernity which is America. Fast-food restaurants let people eat quickly and without planning, without dressing up, without having to make many decisions, and without having to get out of car (Jacobsen and Fritschner,

1991). In the US between 40–50% of the food dollar is spent on food eaten outside of the home and of this 50% is spent in fast-food restaurants. The top four fast-food chains (McDonald's, Burger King, Kentucky Fried Chicken, Pizza Hut) have between them over 32 000 restaurants with combined annual sales of $35 billion US.

> In an industry that has 200 000 separate restaurant companies, McDonald's has 17% of all restaurant visits in the US and 7.3% of all dollars Americans spend on eating out. It controls 20% of fast food market and sells one third of all hamburgers sold by commercial restaurants and one quarter of all french fries.
>
> *Love (1986)*

To remain at the forefront of American consciousness, fast-food chains spend enormous amounts of money on advertising – much of it directed to children. According to Jacobsen and Fritschner (1991) the top eight chains spent $1 billion US on advertising in 1989. McDonald's is the single most advertised brand and in that same year spent $20 million US on Saturday morning television ads aimed at children. Increasingly, commercial tie-ins are used to attract customers – with free plastic figurines from popular culture an especially attractive lure for children. The potential market is of course enormous. Four times out of five when children under 17 years eat out they do so at fast-food restaurants.

The nature of the fast-food enterprise

The phenomenal success of the fast-food restaurants is seen by some critics to be part of a larger and ongoing social evolution. George Ritzer calls this the McDonaldization of society, by which he means the process by which the principles of the fast-food restaurant are coming to dominate more and more sectors of American society as well as of the rest of the world. Ritzer examines fast-food restaurants in a Weberian framework, seeing them as logical successors to the organized rationality of bureaucracies, the work efficiencies of Taylorism and the assembly line methods of Ford. In an increasingly rationalized society, he argues, we come to value efficiency, calculability, predictability and control, all of which are embodied by the modern fast-food operation (Ritzer, 1993).

In Ritzer's words, fast-food restaurants are the most efficient way of getting from a state of being hungry to a state of being full. In North American society efficiency has come to be seen as a virtue, as something to be desired in and of itself. Fast-food restaurants are paeans to efficiency. Every aspect of the operation is designed to maximize output and minimize input with the least expenditure of effort. Anything which wastes time is, by definition, inefficient, so the restaurant is set up for speed; to achieve this, menu items are limited and standardized – so that a customer wishing for a well-done burger or one without the standard 'fixings' causes big problems for the server and probably a long wait for him or herself. In many instances customers are asked to do the work themselves of adding ketchup, relish or whatever to their plain burgers. Having made a purchase, the customer is encouraged to eat quickly and leave. Drive-through windows make the process even more efficient in that the customer leaves before eating – and disposes of their own rubbish afterwards. Efficiency is also the watchword in preparation of fast food menu items. Pre-packaged ingredients preclude time-consuming chopping and peeling operations. Lettuce and cheese for example may arrive pre-shredded. One fast-food chain uses frozen ready-cooked beef in bags which staff simply drop into boiling water. Precise instruction manuals ensure that products are handled in exactly the right way, without unnecessary operations. Paper and cardboard wrappings dispense with the need for dish-washing.

The quest for efficiency, the most impact for the least effort, has been spurred in many sectors by a crunch on scarce resources. Thus efficiency is seen to be identical to cost-effectiveness – the most impact for the least money – and is the basis for Ritzer's second criterion – calculability. In line with the 'bigger is better' philosophy, quantity is seen to be more important than quality. In the fast food business, customers like to know how much they are getting (preferably a lot) for their money (preferably a little). Managers like to know that they are not giving more than they have to. With the aid of technology the supply side has become infinitely quantifiable. Raw ingredients arrive in measured amounts; burger patties weigh exactly the same; french fries are delivered in standard portions; soft drinks are poured by automatic dispensers. Such precise portion control allows for cost control and maintains profitability. From the customer point of view it enables an assessment to be made of value for money, though this is largely illusory. The 'cheap' food bought for a few dollars may consist of a small white bun, 1.6 ounces of meat, a few pennies' worth of potato and a generous helping of flavoured water, sugar and ice. One of the reasons that burger chains initially had a hard time getting established in England was that people were used to much larger quantities of finger-foods, as with the traditional take-away meal of fish and chips.

The third element of Ritzer's McDonaldization process is that of predictability. We no longer like surprises, he says, but prefer conformity to diversity. There are many examples of this tendency in the area of foodways. For example, I have noted elsewhere in this book the relatively limited nature of recipe repertoires. We tend to eat the same things, cooked in the same ways on a fairly regular basis. In working-class England in the 1950s and 1960s one could tell which day of the week it was by what was served for dinner. Experimentation and innovation are self-actualising activities which involve some degree of risk and which are therefore often eschewed in favour of the tried and true. The longing for predictability has also influenced the food supply, as with fruits and vegetables for example, where standardized products are favoured with consequent suppression of variety and, in many instances, flavour. Choosing a restaurant in which to eat out is an inherently unpredictable activity; some of the uncertainty can be removed by referring to a restaurant guide in which someone else has already taken the risk and has spelled out what to expect. No such guide is needed for the fast-food restaurant, which is at the apex of predictability. No matter what time of day, in what city, where in the world – a particular fast-food restaurant chain will serve an identical product. Thus when travelling abroad one need no longer run the risk of being exposed to a different culture, but can seek the reassurance of the familiar food of home.

The last of Ritzer's criteria of rationalization is that of control. In order to bring about efficiency, calculability and predictably, one must be able to exert a great deal of control over a process. That this is exactly what fast-food restaurant chains do has been shown by examples in the foregoing text. To ensure a predictable product fast-food restaurant chains make as many elements of their operations as predictable as possible. Hence the standardization of raw ingredients, the rules for food preparation and the rituals of serving.

Impact of fast food on food habits

The sheer size of the fast-food enterprise guarantees that it has a considerable influence on the eating habits of large segments of the population. On any given day one in five Americans eats in a fast-food restaurant; during the course of a month four out of five Americans will have eaten in a fast-food restaurant. As a result new products, if successful, affect the food habits of millions.

There has been continuing debate over the nutritional value of fast foods. Critics refer to them as 'junk food' while supporters insist that they can be part of a healthy diet. Some companies retain their own nutritionists who produce nutrient profile charts and 'educational' material demonstrating the nutritional virtue of their product. Official food guides tend to relegate them to the category variously known as 'other' or 'extras'. There can be little argument over the fact that most fast foods are high in calories and fat; that this is not particularly problematical in the context of a varied, balanced diet should also be uncontroversial. However, when, as evidence suggest, fast foods become a major dietary component for large numbers of people there may indeed be legitimate health concerns. In addition to high fat contents, fast foods such as french fries are dredged in salt and sugar to give them flavour.

As the industry found that its protestations of being a part of a healthy diet fell on increasingly deaf ears, it began to capitulate to the trend to lower-fat foods. Leaner meat, use of plant oils for frying, low-fat ice-cream and frozen yoghurt, and even salad bars were introduced. Leading magazines in 1991 were full of articles on the new healthier fast foods and the end to artery-clogging burgers. However, the movement was short-lived and by 1993 the same magazines were documenting the trend back to high-calorie, high-fat, large portion size products. Many 'health' lines, such as skinless chicken, had proven to be disastrous. Analysts concluded that people who ate at fast-food restaurants were not interested in health, despite what they might say. McDonald's now has a triple cheeseburger containing 136 g of beef and 540 kcal and is experimenting with a burger containing a half-pound of beef. Domino's pizza chain offer the world's largest pizza, measuring 76 cm and weighing in at 2 kg. Ice-cream manufacturers too are reporting better sales for high-butterfat products. Possible reasons for this revival in the fortunes of high-fat foods include a more accepting social attitude toward weight and a dietary response to the pressures of an economic recession, when people find comfort and reassurance in rich food. Certainly, diet products are no longer in the great vogue they enjoyed in the 1980s and diet books do not dominate the best seller lists as they used to. Nevertheless supermarkets continue to stock and sell low-fat products and some fast-food chains have found a niche selling low-calorie, low-fat food which is baked, grilled and steamed.

Family food habits, cooking skills and grazing

The prime target for fast-food restaurants is the family unit. This makes good commercial sense for as well as enhancing profitability (feeding four or five mouths instead of one) it introduces children to the culture of fast food. Families are increasingly hard-pressed in a fast-paced consumer society to find time for all their desired pursuits. In many two parent families both parents work; single parents often work double shifts or take two jobs to make ends meet. Children are enrolled in endless organized recreational classes and must be transported to and fro. There is little time left to eat – a problem which the fast-food restaurant would seem to solve. The adequacy of this substitution is open to question.

> Do families who eat their suppers at the Colonel's, swinging on plastic seats, or however the restaurant is arranged, say grace before picking up a crispy brown chicken leg? Does dad ask junior what he did today as he remembers he forgot the piccalilli and trots through the crowds to the counter to get some? Does Mom find the atmosphere conducive to asking little Mildred about the problems she was having with third conjugation French verbs, or would it matter since otherwise the family might have been at home chomping down precooked frozen food, warmed in the microwave oven and watching 'Hollywood Squares'.

Ritzer (1993)

However, as Jacobsen and Fritschner observe, fast-food restaurants are remarkably resilient to anything which toddlers can do to them! They are also perceived more and more as places of entertainment. Playground structures and clowns offering face painting attract both the children they are designed for and the parents who are only too grateful to have their offspring distracted, however momentarily.

One consequence of the ready availability of supposedly cheap food outside of the home is a devaluation in the importance of cooking skills. It is difficult to disentangle cause and effect here, though probably they feed off each other. If prepared food is so easily accessible, why bother to learn to cook? If you haven't acquired cooking skills then fast foods are the most efficient answer. Further, the same technologies which have supported the development of the fast-food industry have changed the nature of food preparation in the home. Frozen pre-prepared foods simply need to be re-heated in a microwave oven; dried foods are ready in an instant when hot water is added. The market has moved on from ready-to-bake cake mixes to complete 'gourmet' meals ready to heat and serve. There is even a can of soup available which contains its own re-heating element, activated by the turn of a key.

Fast-food restaurants in North America are commonly open around the clock. People can eat when they want and are no longer confined to traditional mealtimes. Food is thus available on demand. To a generation which has grown up in a culture of fast-food restaurants this is quite normal, and discrete feeding events have become increasingly replaced by the phenomenon known as 'grazing', whereby family members can eat alone at different times to suit their busy schedules. It is therefore not unreasonable to claim that the fast-food restaurant has done its part to contribute to the disruption of family eating practices.

Fast-food culture has also had a devaluing effect on traditional family food events. Parents, too busy or unwilling to stage birthday parties for their children can now hand over responsibility to the local friendly fast-food restaurant. The important social messages encoded in a family birthday celebration risk being overwhelmed by what is in essence a commercial transaction. How long, one wonders, will it be before fast-food weddings catch on or we get fast-food funeral meals for mourners in a hurry?

Fast food in the wider social context

The amount of time devoted to the acquisition and preparation of food has declined as societies have first industrialized and then rationalized. Among hunting and gathering societies the bulk of time is devoted to food procurement. People move to follow the food source or to take advantage of seasonality and food preservation for leaner times is essential. Agriculturalists and pastoralists ensure that a steady food supply is kept to hand and so have to spend less time in food getting. In a modern complex, money-based economy, where a wide variety of foods is available year-round from readily-accessible food depots known as supermarkets, relatively little time is needed for food acquisition. (It is interesting to note however that modern supermarkets co-opt the customer as a willing and unpaid worker in 'hunting' through the shelves and 'gathering' cartloads of groceries. This progress from the full-serve grocery store is presumably a reflection of the search for efficiency previously discussed, although it is doubtful whether standing in endless supermarket queues could be deemed to be efficient – except for the store manager.) Fast-food restaurants and home convenience foods and technologies have diminished further the time needed for food-related activities. The futuristic vision of a meal in a pill no longer seems unreal; indeed, companies involved in the weight-loss industry have already taken great strides down this path with powdered one-package 'meals'.

Fast-food culture has reached into most if not all social organizations. Fast-food outlets are found in schools, hospitals, military bases, airports, train stations and on university campuses. They have formed partnerships with other business sectors in order to take advantage of cross-marketing. Fast-food outlets are found in toy store chains; they sponsor commercial and community events and they have even taken to the road to serve at festive events.

The appearance of fast-food outlets in schools has sparked considerable controversy. The school, as a major agent of secondary socialization, has a potentially great influence on future food habits of students. By endorsing and actually providing fast food fare on the premises schools may be creating conflicts between what is taught as nutrition education and what is practised. Even though it is not yet commonplace for commercial outlets to be sited directly in schools the pressure of the fast food culture has led many school cafeterias to offer similar fare. Fast-food chains have also attempted to develop linkages with schools by promoting student achievement schemes, whereby a pupil earning good grades receives a voucher entitling her to a free burger. Several chains have attempted to establish such a connection between fast food and academic success, including the production of promotional material thinly disguised as 'education'.

The arrival of fast-food outlets in hospitals confronts the health issue even more directly. It has been likened to putting a liquor store in an alcohol dependency unit. If indeed a hospital should be symbolic of health or healing it is ironic that it should provide a local food supply reproducing the very dietary patterns associated with so many of today's chronic diseases.

The global scene: toward cultural homogeneity

Because fast-food restaurants are basically the same from one place to another they are beginning to make cities interchangeable. The same food from the same restaurants is available wherever one goes. One of the consequences of this is a cultural homogeneity which masks or suppresses regional food differences. Even when regional cuisines are acknowledged they are quickly bastardized to meet mainstream tastes, as is illustrated by so-called Mexican fast food wherein the bun is replaced by a taco and the burger has a mild salsa smeared on it. Currently 'Cajun' sauces are being used to do the same for Louisiana cuisine.

Fast-food restaurants developed in the United States and it is there that they continue to enjoy a growing hegemony. However, in the constant search for new markets fast-food chains have increasingly looked overseas. Their ready spread into Canada is fairly understandable given the geographic proximity and cultural dominance of the US, but McDonald's is also the biggest restaurant chain in Germany, England, Australia and Japan. The largest McDonald's opened in Beijing in 1992 surpassing an existing Kentucky Fried Chicken franchise. World media attention was accorded to McDonald's when it opened a franchise in Moscow, and it was reported that Muscovites lined up for hours for the privilege of paying a good part of their wages for a burger and fries. The opening up of the former Eastern bloc to Western style capitalist enterprise holds the promise of a giant new market for fast food.

In expanding into foreign markets fast-food chains have on the whole been most successful when they have maintained the basic American menu; attempts to adapt to other national cuisines have failed. In Japan, where beef was previously little eaten, the hamburger was marketed with revolutionary audacity, with claims that such a diet would eventually make the Japanese people taller, whiter and blonder. Experience in Germany also showed that despite initially differing food habits consumers would accept an American food system which did not try to compromise with local tastes. Instead, compromises to foreign markets have tended to be on the physical environments of the restaurants rather than on the food itself.

Subsequently, the influence of fast-food culture has been felt in the traditional realms of European cuisine. Much to general surprise, fast-food croissanteries have taken root in Paris. American fast food is not alone in its global pretensions. Harry Ramsden's, the only fish and chip shop to appear on the British stock market, is also looking at establishing an overseas presence. Shops are planned for Jeddah in Saudi Arabia and in Singapore and negotiations are under way for an Australian franchise.

Resistance and backlash

While fast-food restaurants have made eating out an affordable activity and have fitted in well to fast-paced lifestyles, not everyone has welcomed them with open arms. In Europe, they have been the focus of protests and even riots by critics who viewed them as a form of American cultural imperialism and as being unsuited to old world settings and values.

Recent public concern with environmental issues has also forced the fast-food industry into a defensive position. Fast-food restaurants use millions of tons of packaging which is discarded within minutes of the food being consumed. Much of this non-biodegradable waste ends up in landfill sites. Consumer protests eventually led to replacement of styrofoam packaging by card, the reduction of paper napkin size and the limited introduction of refillable coffee cups – measures for which the industry now takes full credit as environmentally responsible corporate citizens. Destruction of rainforests in Latin America for conversion to beef cattle ranches provided the impetus for a consumer boycott of McDonald's in the 1980s. Although it now claims to use no beef which has been raised on land converted from rainforest, as the world's biggest single purchaser of beef McDonald's has a global influence on agricultural and land-use policies.

The health lobby appears to have met with mixed success. Fast-food chains have shown an ability and willingness to provide lower-fat products and additional menu items such as juices and salads. However, they are quick to drop those items which are not commercially popular and economically profitable. This provides a dilemma for nutrition educators; should they continue to try to persuade fast-food merchants to find acceptable healthier items or should they try to convince people to make less use of fast-food restaurants? Recent trends suggest that both of these are going to be difficult tasks.

EKIBEN: JAPANESE RAILWAY FOOD

Ekiben is a food phenomenon which illustrates a very different aspect to mass feeding than the burger and pizza culture previously discussed. In Japanese, **Eki** means station and **ben** is an abbreviation of **bentou** which means lunch box or meal prepared for eating out. Therefore, Ekiben is a bentou sold at a station; because Ekiben was developed for the convenience of railway passengers in the 19th century the term refers exclusively to railway stations, though bentou, or box lunches are widely available and are taken to school, office and factory, to the theatre or on trips to the countryside. There are probably over 1600 varieties of Ekiben sold to commuters, tourists and travellers at Japan's 5000 railway stations. An estimated 12 million Ekiben are sold each day at station kiosks and by roving platform vendors. Ekiben has been called the most sophisticated fast food in the world.

The word bentou first appeared in the literature in the 16th century, referring to meals prepared for eating out. In the 18th century such meals would be prepared for the Kabuki theatre where play performances could last up to 10 hours and there was no restaurant. Patrons bought their own lunch to eat during the intermission, or could buy bentou from outside catering services. Bentou prepared for the Kabuki theatre were known as Maku-no-uchi bentou which meant 'bentou to eat during the time when the stage curtain was hanging down'. One typical pattern of Maku-no-uchi bentou was a three-layered wooden box containing familiar and widely acceptable foods. The top layer was packed with items such as cooked shrimp, grilled fish or fish cake, small sushi or thick omelette; the middle layer contained well-seasoned cooked vegetables and pickles; the bottom layer contained white rice with sesame seeds or seasoned rice, sometimes moulded into one-bite size pieces or into the shape of leaves or flowers. The Maku-no-uchi bentou remained popular for eating out not only at the theatre but also on picnics and journeys and is therefore considered to be the prototype of the modern Ekiben.

Individual bento were distributed at social occasions where there were too many guests for each to be served personally. The practicality of this custom led, in Kyoto, to widespread use of lunchbox meals as a substitute for home cooking. In hard times, soldiers got a hinomaru bento, a 'lunchbox of the rising sun' which consisted of a red plum on a bed of white rice, symbolising the Japanese flag (Terzani and Wolf, 1987).

History of Ekiben

The first passenger railroad was established between Shinbashi (now a part of Tokyo) and Yokohama in 1872. Although opinions differ, the most common view is that the first Ekiben was of the Omusubi type (see below) and was sold at Utsunomiya station in the Kanto region in 1885. This original Ekiben comprised two rice balls packed around pickled plums, sprinkled with sesame salt and wrapped in a bamboo leaf. Recent evidence leads some authorities to believe that an unspecified bentou was sold at Ueno station (now a part of Tokyo) in 1883.

Ekiben were at first simple enough to meet the modest requirements of most passengers. However, travel has always been viewed as an 'occasion' for many Japanese people and the more elaborate Maku-no-uchi bentou appeared at Koube station in the Chugoku region as early as 1888. The first train dining car was introduced in 1889 but it served only Western meals and was designed specifically for foreign travellers who were not accustomed to Japanese food. Now, rail travellers can enjoy both Western and Japanese food in the dining car as well as Ekiben eaten at their own seats.

Bentou outlets are found in a variety of settings in a modern town; in parks, baseball stadiums and in front of office buildings. They may be small shops operated by a large chain store and supplied everyday from the central kitchen, or the 'take-out' service associated with a restaurant. Renowned restaurants offer very high quality (and high priced) bentou.

There is a significant difference between bentou sold in town and Ekiben sold at railway stations. Common lunch bentou are prepared to meet the preferences of the regular Japanese customer, but Ekiben are designed to feature local speciality foods. Travellers who are curious to taste different local specialities may choose routes accordingly, and Japan Railways issues a guide to what Ekiben are available at which stations in which seasons and for what cost.

Large city department stores hold special Ekiben fairs, at which Ekiben from stations nationwide are sold. These are always extremely successful; people may buy a particular Ekiben as a reminder of a past trip taken or to recall the tastes of their home town. Modern day Ekiben are sophisticated and diverse; the food itself is sometimes surprising, and the inventive containers range from simple and plain to elegant and whimsical.

Description of Ekiben

At first Ekiben were of two basic types, common bentou and speciality bentou. The former was a simple combination of rice and some other ingredient; the latter would use a special recipe representing a particular locality. Now, the wide variety of Ekiben can be described as belonging to one of five main categories. **Maku-no-uchi** was traditionally served at theatres as described above. It might be characterized as a sort of variety pack, and commonly features a regimented, crisply geometric display with a carefully balanced colour scheme (Kamekura, Bosker and Watanabe, 1989). **Donburi** is a typical light lunch meal originally served in a porcelain bowl called a Donburi. It comprises cooked rice covered with seasoned ingredients such as meat, fish and vegetables. There are many varieties of recipe and container. For example, Kama-meshi is cooked in a pan called a Kama. Oyster Kama-meshi would then be tasty rice with oyster cooked in a Kama. Popular Donburi- type Ekiben include Unagi (grilled eel), sukiyaki, chicken, oyster and scallop.

Sushi Ekiben feature seafood. However, unlike at popular sushi bars where fresh raw seafood is used, in Ekiben it is acidified with vinegar, a traditional method used prior to the advent of refrigeration. Sugar may be added to the rice to help preserve the product and, in some instances, sushi dishes actually benefit from being left for 24 hours before consumption. Still, the seafood used should be caught in the vicinity of the station selling it; common varieties are salmon, yellowfin horse mackerel, red sea bream, pacific saury, tiger puffer and ayu – a Japanese river fish. Masu No Sushi sold at Toyama station features river trout (masu) and is one of the most popular Ekiben in Western Japan. **Omusubi** is the most simple and inexpensive bentou. Rice is pressed into a spherical or triangular shape and ingredients such as grilled salmon or pickled plum are stuffed in the centre and wrapped by black seaweed. A miscellaneous category embraces local specialities. For example, in a region famous for producing high-quality noodles, a noodle bentou will be found at the local train station. The cooking method itself may be the speciality. So, squid bentou is prepared by stuffing rice into the body of the squid and then cooking it. Sandwiches are also popular as a light Ekiben.

In addition to these basic categories, there are also a number of typical cooking styles for bentou. Kama-meshi, as mentioned above utilizes cooked rice with other ingredients in a Kama-shaped pan. Tooge No Kama-meshi from Yokokawa station is considered to be one of the finest of Japan's Ekiben. Two brands of high-quality rice are cooked, lightly flavoured and then topped with chicken, shiitake mushrooms, burdock and apricot. No preservative or artificial flavouring is added. This was the first Ekiben to use a pottery container. Tori-meshi is rice cooked in chicken stock, covered by chicken pieces cooked in various ways. Tori-meshi is sold at Takasaki station in the northern Kanto region. Kani-meshi is seasoned rice covered by crab flakes. Cha-meshi is seasoned rice with a green tea flavour. Okowa uses seasoned glutinous rice. Unagi-meshi is rice covered by charcoal-grilled eel.

The name of the Ekiben generally reflects speciality local ingredients. A Japanese guide entitled 'Topography of Delicious Ekiben' details the Ekiben available at stations in the eight regions of Japan (Kodansha, 1991). Photographs are accompanied by descriptions of the food and current prices, which range from 350 to 1200 yen, with sushi Ekiben being the most expensive. Each region of the long narrow country has its own range of typical foods and cooking methods. Tables 10.1 and 10.2 show regional variations in Ekiben by type and speciality, while Figure 10.1 locates the regions geographically.

Because of the emphasis on freshness in Japanese cookery the concept of seasonality is an important one. Some Ekiben reflect seasonal changes in the availability of fresh ingredients. For example, Tako-meshi Ekiben is sold at Mihara station only from May to October when octopus is in season. In late autumn Ekiben here feature matsutake mushroom rice; during the winter, oyster rice is the signature preparation.

Table 10.1 Variation in types of Ekiben predominant in different geographical regions of Japan

Area of Japan	Most common type of Ekiben (%)				
	Maku-no-uchi	Donburi	Sushi	Omusubi	Other
Hokkaido Island	15	55	25	02	03
Tohoku	38	50	05	02	05
Kanto and Tokyo	60	30	15	03	02
Honsyu Centre	10	20	60	10	-
Tokai and Kinki	20	12	60	04	04
Chugoku	10	30	60	-	-
Shikoku Island	50	-	50	-	-
Kyusyu Island	63	25	12	-	-

Table 10.2 Sample Ekiben specialities in geographical regions of Japan

Hokkaido Island	Salmon, crab, scallop, clam, herring
Tohoku	Scallop, mackerel, sea urchin, abalone, wheat noodle, mushroom
Kanto and Tokyo	Chestnut, chicken, plum, eel
Honsyu Centre	Guinea fowl, salmon, red sea bream
Tokai and Kinki	Beef, shrimp, crab, saury, sea trout, takana green leaf, persimmon leaf
Chugoku	Octopus, sardine, conger, ayu, tiger puffer, flying fish, pine mushroom
Shikoku Island	Ayu, bonito, mackerel
Kyusyu Island	Spiced cod roe, chicken, pork, aquilla

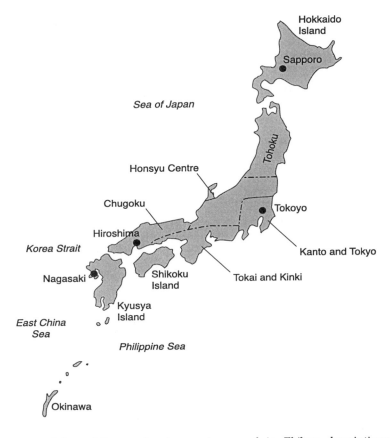

Figure 10.1 Map of Japan showing regions used in Ekiben descriptions. 1, Hokkaido Island; 2, Honsyu Centre; 3, Tohuku; 4, Kanto and Tokyo; 5, Tokai and Kinki; 6, Shikoku Island; 7, Kyusya Island; 8, Chugoku

Fast food and aesthetics

'If in the West the label "fast food" conjures up images of uniformly drab, mass-produced, and uninspired menus, in Japan Ekiben stands for foods with a vibrantly regional inflection, dished up with wildly inventive local color' (Kamekura, Bosker and Watanabe, 1989). North American fast food is designed for a car-dependent society; a burger can be readily eaten with one hand while the other remains on the steering wheel. Everything about it, from the ingredients to the packaging emphasizes standardization and uniformity. There are no surprises; it is dull. In contrast, Japanese fast food for the train is remarkable for its diversity. Each station offers up a unique product taking advantage of local foods and seasonal changes. The food is served in visually appealing containers of different materials including bamboo, ceramics and wood as well as plastic. There are even containers shaped like golf balls and tennis rackets to be found at stations that service resort areas.

In small town stations the production of Ekiben may be a family concern, whereas in larger cities it is a commercial business. Large numbers of people use the trains, and it is assumed that approximately 1% of passengers will buy Ekiben, requiring even small stations to provide about 300 Ekiben per day (K. Wani, personal communication). Except for simple processes such as packing and moulding of rice which may be mechanized in larger operations, Ekiben are usually assembled by hand. About two-thirds of the day's production is completed for the morning trade; how much more is produced for the afternoon depends on the morning sales and what is left-over. The time at which the Ekiben was assembled must legally be displayed on the packaging. Since all products should be sold at the end of the day, sales managers devote considerable effort to forecasting sales each day.

Whereas the burger represents the utilitarian ethos of America, Ekiben reproduce the aesthetic values associated with Japanese food and art. Visual qualities of food are as important to the Japanese as the taste of the food itself. Formal meals may be miniature edible masterpieces while even home cooking pays attention to form, shape and colour. Small pieces of food are neatly arranged with decorative garnishes. Ekiben food itself, despite being mass-produced, can appear as a work of art. Sometimes compartments are used to keep food items separate but often the various ingredients are attractively arranged in exquisite free-form or to form patterns of harmonious colours. The box for SL bento from Sapporo station is divided into an upper compartment with several sections that resemble train windows and which contain local specialities; the lower rice compartment has 'wheels' made of dried seaweed embedded in it, or rice wheels wrapped in seaweed strips. Examples of Ekiben are illustrated in Figures 10.2 and 10.3.

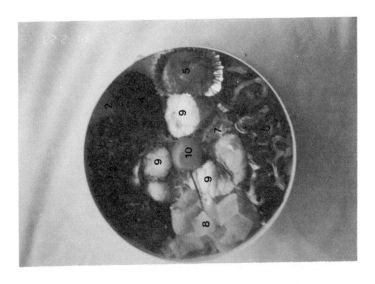

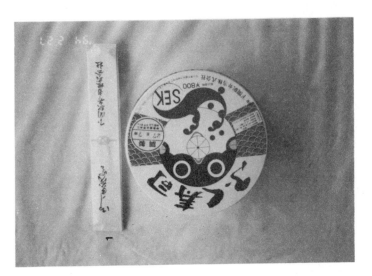

Figure 10.2 Fugu-sushi bentou sold at Shinshimonoseki railway station. 1, chopstick; 2, base layer of garnish, acidified rice; 3, seasoned seaweed; 4, Shiitake mushroom; 5, squid with sea-urchin sauce; 6, skin of tiger puffer; 7, thin sliced egg-film; 8, pickled radish; 9, three pieces of cooked tiger puffer; 10, cherry.

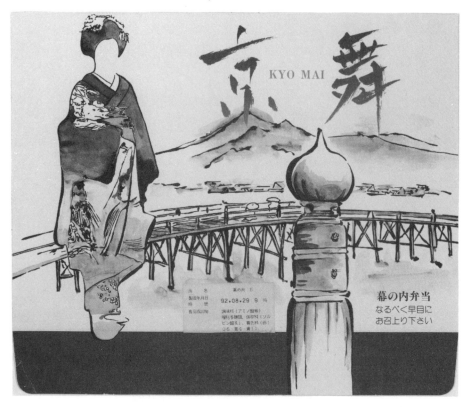

Figure 10.3 Ekiben packaging showing product information. The label shows: 1. The name of the product, MAKU NO UCH (B is an abbreviation for bentou); 2. The date and time of manufacture (92, 08, 29; 9.^{00} (morning)). 3. Food additives – seasoning (amino acids, etc.), polysaccharides, preservatives (K-sorbate), colour (red no. 1, no. 6, yellow 4, blue 1).

Ekiben containers are an art form in themselves. The exterior wrapping or box decoration can be used to depict the region from which the Ekiben comes, the type of food within, or the origin of the dish. A pastoral scene or depiction of an event from some legend are as likely as the drawing of a lobster illustrating how it is caught. One practical Ekiben box has drawings and descriptions of traditional games for the passenger to while away their time. Chochin Bento is served in a lantern-style container reminiscent of the famous paper lanterns or chochin of the Kanagawa region. Okayama, known for its chestnuts (kuri), sells Kuri Okowa in a chestnut-shaped box. Similarly, Hotate Fuki-Yose is served in a scallop-shaped container. Some containers have additional uses; one has a cut-out of a traditional 'moon-face', which can be used as a mask; others can be turned into piggy-banks. Complex Ekiben contain several courses arranged in layers in a series of pull-out trays. Hama Gozen is a two-tiered Ekiben sold at Shin-Yokohama station. The wooden container is first tied with a red and white ceremonial rope and then wrapped in a cloth printed with flowers and turtles. The top layer has various foods, neatly arranged; the bottom layer holds rice in the shape of a fan, and sonomono.

Myth and legend

Tanabata is a festival held every July 7th, a day when young girls write their wishes on paper strips and hang them from bamboo branches. Sendai city is known for its elaborate Tanabata celebration. Kokeshi, a wooden doll, is the most popular souvenir of the area. The local Ekiben for Sendai station is known as Tanabata Kokeshikko and comprises chicken teriyaki, kamaboko with plum flavour and boiled chestnuts on rice, in a ceramic container decorated with a stylized doll's face.

Kiyohime No Ichiya Sushi from Gobou station is inspired by a love story in which Kiyohime, the daughter of a wealthy merchant, followed Anjin, the monk she loved, bringing him what she thought was the most delicious of all foods, the nare-sushi of Kishu. Local mackerel is salted and pressed for one night and then wrapped in bamboo leaf with rice. It is presented in a beautiful rectangular container of bamboo wood and leaves, wrapped in a decorative paper wrapper depicting Kiyohime with her hair streaming behind her.

These examples illustrate the vitality and beauty it is possible to bring to fast food.

FLY ME – I'M HUNGRY

We serve eight million passengers a year and it is a no-win situation. We must constantly change to cope with different tastes and demands.

Airline Food Survey (1993)

As air travel has become an increasingly common, even mundane, part of routine life, more and more people are moved about in pressurized tubes 30 000 feet above the Earth. There were an estimated 1170 million passengers on domestic and international airlines in 1992. Whether they travel for business or pleasure these customers share one thing in common – they need to eat. Airline food is in some ways simply a special case of institutionalized feeding. However, the challenge of mass feeding in such constrained conditions is a considerable one; one which creates its own peculiar food culture.

So what purpose does food service on aircraft serve? Obviously the answer is more than a simple utilitarian one. It would not be unreasonable to suppose that food in the air fulfils a range of similar functions and carries similar meanings to those encoded in foodways everywhere. There is of course the need to provide food for sustenance when 'normal' meal-times occur during the flight and when a considerable flight time is involved. However, this does not explain the felt need to serve meals on flights of short duration; in some cases the meal service is uncomfortably hurried so as to fit it in between reaching cruising altitude and final descent. Some airlines cope with this by providing a snack instead of a meal, or by providing snack food at the terminal prior to departure. (Lufthansa passengers can even fill a snack bag at the terminal and take it on board with them.) In any case there seems to be an expectation that some sort of food will be served.

Meeting passengers' hunger needs is only one goal of airline food service; others are perhaps less obvious. For example, the routinized appearance of drinks, snacks and meals marks the passage of time in an environment where few other temporal markers are available. Food also relieves boredom and monotony on long flights – providing captive passengers with something to do. Related to this, from the airline perspective, food service helps to keep passengers in their seats and out of the way of the cabin crew, minimizing disruptions in the smooth operation of the overall in-flight service and allowing the crew to concentrate on doing their jobs. But perhaps most importantly food service conveys all the messages normally expected of a host catering to guests. The idea of the passenger as guest is one which many airlines attempt to emphasize; in Air Canada it is reflected in the designation of economy fare passengers as 'Hospitality Class'.

Eating is a social occasion. On aeroplane flights passengers are seated usually next to complete strangers. While some gregarious souls strike up conversations which last from take-off to touch-down, others utter not a word to their neighbours. The serving of the meal, the lifting of the tray cover to discover the secrets beneath, the first taste of the food (whether approving or otherwise), the awkwardness of opening the plastic wrappers around the utensils or organising the food tray so that one can actually eat without spilling everything – all are invitations to make conversational remarks – to acknowledge the fellow passenger as someone who is basically sharing your food. Even if conversations are not pursued one is reassured that one belongs here; that there is a thread of common humanity.

Thus airline food service does indeed fulfil biocultural functions, reassuring us that despite being in a pressurized tube 30 000 feet in the air, social conventions are still in effect. In further examining airline food culture and food service, two intertwined themes seem to stand out; those of choice and social status. Minor themes include aesthetics and nutrition or health.

Choice

From the point of view of the airlines as food providers, choice is constrained by practical considerations of space, weight, time and cost. From the passengers' perspective there are major restrictions on their choice of foods, of when to eat and of dining companions. The provider thus exerts much more control over the feeding situation than is normal. Some airlines are sensitive to this issue and are diligent about restoring passenger choice – or at least the illusion of choice. The most common way to do this is via multiple menu options; commonly two alternatives are offered in Economy Class while up to four choices may be available to passengers in First Class seats. In some instances there may be a degree of choice over when to eat rather than submitting to a mass feeding frenzy at a pre-ordained time. Many airlines provide menus to passengers, sometimes very elaborate ones, which provide an illusion of restaurant catering and fine dining.

Menu choices are extended for those passengers declaring special needs. A range of meals designed to meet medical prescriptions, religious requirements and cultural preferences may be available through pre-ordering. The knowing passenger may utilize this system to obtain different meal choices even though not having any personal medical or cultural food restrictions.

Airlines contacted by this author provided from 8 to 30 special diets or variations thereof (Table 10.3). Some were common to airlines around the world; others reflected specific regional food cultures. For example, Air India offers a strict Jain diet. The 'Very strict Indian vegetarian meal' offered by Cathay Pacific excludes root vegetables, ginger, garlic, onion and potato. Vegetarian alternatives were perhaps the most common in the cultural category, with some airlines differentiating between 'Western' and 'Asian' vegetarian. In the religious category, Kosher meals were provided by nearly all airlines surveyed. Common medical diets included low-salt, low-calorie and diabetic adaptations. Saudi Arabia Airlines has developed a special meal for blind passengers. Braille menus indicate the layout and make-up of the meal, and specially selected foods and utensils are used to make it easier for blind passengers to manage (Aviation Week, 1993).

Some airlines do not provide certain special meals because they cannot guarantee compliance with dietary prescriptions. For example, Air Canada does not list nut-free meals due to difficulty in guaranteeing that peanut oil or derivatives have not been used in preparation. A similar rationale is given for not listing allergy-sensitive meals. Allergy and gluten-free diets are not provided by KLM Dutch Airlines because in certain parts of the world the ingredients and the facilities for their preparation are not readily available.

Table 10.3 Special meals available on world airlines

(Western) Vegetarian
Vegetarian – Lacto-ovo
Vegan
Oriental Vegetarian
Indian (Asian) Vegetarian
Very Strict Indian Vegetarian
Kosher
Moslem
Hindu (non-vegetarian)
Jain
Moslem (non-Halal)
Fish
Fruit Plate
Nutri-Action
Infant Food
Junior Food
Child Meal
Low cholesterol
Diabetic
Bland/light low fibre/ ulcer
Low-protein
Gluten-free
High-fibre
Low-fat
Low-sodium
Low-calorie
Liquid diet
Cholesterol-free
Cardiovascular diet
Non-lactose
Low-purine
High-protein
Acid meal

Cathay Pacific prints a small pamphlet for staff to enable them to respond to passenger requests. Special meals available from the airline are listed with a brief description and special notes. For example under the descriptor 'Indian vegetarian' staff are informed that 'This is a vegetarian meal cooked in an Indian style and does not include any meat, fish, egg, game or seafood. Dairy products such as milk, cream and yoghurt will be used. Meals are always available as a regular menu choice on the full itinerary of CX 751/750', and are further reminded that 'This meal is ordered by the great majority of Hindus who cannot eat meat or fish. Most Hindus require this meal and the passenger's special need should be identified and accurately coded.'. Kosher meals are 'prepared according to Jewish law and are bought from reputable manufacturers. There are several brands used in our network and the best available product in each port will be uplifted. From Hong Kong a frozen product is offered and 24 hours notice of request is therefore vital'.

Food items preferred by passengers vary, as would be expected, from airline to airline depending partially on the routes served. Thus Cathay Pacific finds Asian noodle dishes to be popular while Air Jamaica scores with calaloo and codfish for breakfast. Air India reports that Indian cuisine is popular with all passengers; even foreigners prefer to have Indian curries. For an international clientele, steaks seem to be popular while for First Class passengers caviar and other luxury products are in demand. Airlines also discover that certain foods are not acceptable or popular and that tastes change. Cheese and butter are not big items on Asian routes; nor are lamb, mutton or cold soups. Passengers with Air Jamaica reject turkey slices. Lufthansa found that pork, which was very popular a few years ago is now hardly accepted.

Another aspect of choice is the use of menu cycles by which airlines attempt to provide sufficient variety for regular travellers. Air Canada divides Canada into four sections each with different menu cycles, so that passengers don't receive the same food on both the outward and return journey. Menus may change as frequently as each week on short-haul European flights, monthly on high-frequency routes and in First Class, and quarterly or seasonally on longer haul, less popular routes.

Usually all passengers eat at approximately the same time at the discretion of the airline. Commonly, especially in Business and First Class, cold sandwiches and other snacks are available on request and in addition to the hot meal. To allow for more passenger choice, Air Canada offers a 'Flex meal' in Business Class. This is a cold plate available at any time during the flight. The future of airline food service may lie in finding ways of allowing passengers more control over when they eat.

Other factors which commonly influence airlines in their food service choices are passenger preferences, convenience, cost, passenger demography, local availability and seasonality, the ability of contract kitchens, origin and destination of flights, and flight duration. Galley space and heating procedures on aircraft are also mentioned, as are lifestyle and nutritional trends. KLM Royal Dutch Airlines use what they call a food concept. The guidelines are departure time, flying time, day or night flight, arrival time and galley space, as well as route service-specific. Passenger preferences are ascertained in a number of ways, the most common of which are surveys, tray left-over audits and feedback from flight attendants. Some airlines hold customer forums or do focus group testing or have a customer advisory board which allows passengers a chance to be involved in product development.

Status

Food and food service on airlines serves or reflects sharp differentiations in attributed social status. This is evident in contrasting First and/or Business Class with Economy or Hospitality class. There are differences in the actual foods and meals served, the number of choices, in the manner of serving and in the aesthetics of the meal service. Frequently the class distinction is marked by a physical separation of First Class from other passengers. First Class passengers have their own food servers who do not attend to the lesser mortals at the back of the plane.

The menu card

Most airlines provide menu cards for their passengers. These vary from the plain to the elaborate and immediately portray the status dimension of airline food. First Class menu cards are typically larger in size, contain more elaborate inserts and are printed on better quality paper or card. Often, there are no printed menus for Economy Class. Similar differences hold for the wine list, which is more often a separate piece in First Class. The First Class wine list for Air Canada describes a selection of champagnes and fine wines together with facsimiles of the wine labels; Business Class has the description without the label facsimiles; Hospitality Class passengers are asked 'White or red?' by the cabin crew. The First Class menu of British Airways announces that it is '..a member of La Confrèrie de la Chaine des Rotisseurs – the world's oldest and most important gastronomical society, founded in 1248 and granted a Royal Charter in 1610.' It offers long-standing traditions of comfort, elegance and hospitality for the discerning traveller.

The food itself

The more expensive the ticket, the more extensive the menu. First Class passengers are offered menus with a greater number of courses or food items on them, with more choices of main course and in many instances with choices in other courses too. This is well illustrated by the sample menus reproduced in Table 10.4.

More expensive foods are typically offered as hor's d'oeuvres while other courses show less differentiation. Smoked salmon, lobster terrine and caviar appear on the First Class menus of many airlines. One American airline commented that First Class and Business Class passengers received larger portions.

Manner of serving

Options for food presentation and serving are limited. Pre-assembled meal trays are common in Economy Class. The hot component of the meal is held in metal heating cabinets and added to a standard meal tray at the time of serving. In First Class, trolley service is more common, recreating to the limited degree possible on an aeroplane, restaurant practices and distracting attention from the mass feeding nature of the enterprise. Precise graduation of status sensibilities is demonstrated by Lufthansa, where First Class has a cart service, Business Class has tray service for the main meal and cart service for cheese and dessert and Economy Class has a tray-only service.

Table 10.4 Dinner Menus from VARIG airlines

Economy[1]	Executive[2]	First Class[3]
Roll & butter	Roll & butter	Hot & cold canapes
	Bon Gourmet plate	Caspian Sea caviar Salmon fillet/ trout mousse Chicken Neva style
		Watercress soup
Duckling 'Balotine' with corn sprout & walnut	Veal steak	Grilled sirloin steak
Mixed skewer	Seafood Maryland	Grilled seafood skewer
Vegetables in butter Rice Valenciennes style	Broccoli menagere Oyster plant au gratin Berny potatoes Gnocci	Spring vegetables Stuffed potatoes Rice, Italian style Mutton Medaillons Gnocci
	Mixed salad	Mixed salad
Quindin (fruit)	Fruit plate with cheese French pastry Chocolate	Cheese-board Fruit basket
Brazilian coffee	Brazilian coffee	Brazilian coffee

[1]Flight reference 2-1804-1J
[2]Flight reference EX-3-1407-1JB
[3]Flight reference 4-1804-1JB (RG/JAL)

Nutrition and health

Concerns in this area are mostly related to special diets though airlines are acknowledging that many of their passengers are becoming more health conscious. Health considerations are reflected in the introduction of 'lifestyle' choices by some airlines. British Airways Club World and World Traveller menus include 'Well-Being Options'. These are identified, with a logo, as 'an alternative dining style that is light, well balanced and easily digested. The dishes are vegetarian and low in salt, sugar and dairy products and are made from quality ingredients.'

While some airlines have their own in-house catering operation many contract with food service companies. In either case there are usually guidelines or qualified dietetic advisers to ensure that special meals meet requirements. As part of a Lufthansa catering series, a 63-page booklet on special meals is available to airline staff to help them present an 'important part of the in-flight service in a convincing and informative manner'. The guide contains colour plates and descriptions of two examples of each special meal. Each example includes a photograph of a First Class item, a hot meal, a cold meal, and a hot and cold breakfast. The narrative identifies the meal type and either a brief descriptor of the meal or who it is intended for. (Gluten-free meal: 'meal for those allergic to gluten'; Fish meal: 'Meal mainly of fish, shellfish and crustaceans'). There then follows a statement of the principles of the diet ('without meat'; 'fresh basic products, high nutritional value'), cooking methods (everything permitted with exception of frying and deep-fat frying) and a list of 'Sundry Items' including breads, drinks, condiments, dressings and sweeteners. Finally, a literal description of the photographed samples is given.

Air Canada provides its flight crews with ingredient lists for dishes so that passenger concerns regarding allergies, religious proscriptions and other food avoidances can easily be checked.

Aesthetics

In the name of convenience and practicality airlines make extensive use of plastic moulded dishes and trays. One of the attractions of a now defunct Canadian airline, Wardair, was meal service (for all passengers) using real china plates and cups. On Thai Airlines, in First Class a special Thai ceramic set, hand painted with gold and five colours is used to serve Thai food. Otherwise glasses, chinaware, silver cutlery, linen napkins and tablecloth are used. In Economy Class it is melamine, stainless steel cutlery, and paper napkins.

The flowering of aesthetic values is, however, best represented by the humble menu card. A menu for Cathay Pacific's Marco Polo Business Class (Hong Kong to Tokyo flight) comes in a full colour, large format.

The card cover design in rich orange and brown tones depicts alchemist motifs, and is entitled *'The elements of Nature'*. One almost expects to find an art gallery catalogue within. The inside cover has a statement (in English) that: 'Cathay Pacific's philosophy has always been to blend the best and most harmonious aspects of East and West. This menu is one of a series depicting the five Elements of Nature that, in Chinese religious beliefs, are symbolized by colours, directions, seasons and living creatures related to Water, Metal, Wood, Fire and Earth. These five elements, like our service today, are a wonderful source of refreshment, nourishment, comfort and pleasure'. Further text describes the history of metal and concludes with the invitation 'As you lift your fork today, consider the role metal plays in our lives'. Here we see acknowledgement of the cultural nature of food. Folded inside this cover is a smaller card of similar design, but containing the drinks and wine list, which appears to be standard for a number of flights. Descriptions of the wines are given. The list is in both Chinese and English. Inside this again, and bound to the whole by a cord, is a fine paper stock insert which contains the actual menu in Chinese, Japanese and English.

A sample First Class menu comes in an even larger format than the Business Class. The card cover is white, with an elegant small photographic reproduction and bearing the legend 'First' on the cover. The inside cover discusses changes in travel wrought by modern jetliners and the efforts of Cathay Pacific to keep alive the 'elusive joy of travel', which is accomplished in part by 'creating in-flight menus that reflect in their own way those same international and Asian influences'. A fine, embossed paper leaf is next, followed by an inside card containing the menu in Chinese, Japanese and English. The card stock has faint watermark like illustrations of tureens, cups and water jugs.

Other airline menus feature reproductions of original paintings. The Brazilian carrier, VARIG uses botanical paintings of Amazon flora with a full description of the painting and artist on the back cover.

Airline food and culture

While some airlines make an effort to reflect the culture of their country in the food which they serve, others pride themselves on an international kitchen. A middle course is fairly popular, which is to offer feature meals on certain dedicated routes, though this is more to accommodate passenger demographics than to showcase cultural dishes.

Air Jamaica does make a particular effort to showcase ethnic cuisine. Jerked chicken is served as an appetizer on First Class flights to New York and Philadelphia. Curried beef or chicken is offered in Economy Class on New York flights. Calaloo, codfish and fried dumplings, bammy or festival with fried plantain is usually served on Miami breakfast flights. Local desserts such as sweet potato pudding are also used.

Cathay Pacific serves predominantly Asian food – Chinese, Japanese, Indian, Thai; while VARIG features Brazilian coffee. Lufthansa has destination feature meals on both outward and homebound intercontinental flights (for example, Japanese, Mexican, Korean), with a specific aim to make passengers familiar with the local cuisine of their destination. Similarly, intercontinental flights also feature a German speciality to make the international passenger familiar with German cuisine. In order to make passengers aware of other cuisines, Air India organizes food festivals on various routes.

The origin and destination of flights is an important factor in food service for many airlines. While they may not showcase their own country's cuisine they do want to ensure that their passengers find the food acceptable and enjoyable. Air Canada makes several arrangements of this type. It will provide an 'oriental meal' for groups of ten or more who pre-book it. On First Class flights to Europe there is a choice of 'regional cuisine' designed to reflect the cultural flavour of Great Britain, France and Germany. On Caribbean flights a strong preference for chicken is catered to. Thai Airlines demonstrates cultural sensitivity by not offering pork on any Middle Eastern routes.

SUMMARY

Over the last 30 years or so, fast food has come to play a dominant role in the food systems of industrialized countries and, increasingly in the developing world; in doing so it has influenced the eating habits of millions of people. Aided by technological innovation fast food is a reflection of, and a response to, the complex, harried lifestyles which typify urban living in many parts of the world. Ritzer (1993) points out that fast-food restaurants have become victims of their own success. Positioned to provide cheap food quickly and efficiently they are no longer cheap, fast or efficient. After waiting in line for 5 or 10 minutes a family of four can pay $20 for a single meal. The experience of fast-food dining is one which promotes anomie and social disjuncture. It attracts with its promise of fun and efficiency, but the fun is short-lived and the efficiency is largely illusory.

The fast-food industry has a major impact on global food and agricultural systems, benefiting from and contributing to continuing delocalization of diets and increasing homogeneity in food habits. However, providing food on a large scale does not necessarily have to lead to sameness and dullness. Japanese railway box meals, Ekiben, demonstrate how aesthetic and gastronomic quality can be preserved in a mass feeding enterprise. Ekiben are prepared fresh each day, utilize local and seasonal ingredients and are artfully and attractively presented. Both Ekiben and burger-and-fries mirror the values of the society in which they exist, the contrast providing an instructive example of the biocultural meaning of food.

Airlines are faced with the challenge of feeding thousands of passengers under demanding conditions. While taking advantage of some of the same technologies that serve the fast-food industry, air carriers have, on the whole, strived to maintain the values and expectations associated with the 'proper meal'. Passenger choice is a key element in food service which, to a greater or lesser degree, reinforces the social status symbolism of food.

FURTHER READING

Three different aspects of the fast-food industry are considered by the main authors cited in this chapter. Ritzer (1993) places fast food in a sociological context; Love (1986) provides an in-depth exploration of the life and times of one fast-food company; Jacobsen and Fritschner (1993) offer a consumer guide to the nutritional value of fast-food products.

Kamekura, Bosker and Watanabe (1989) is a source of stunningly beautiful photographs of Ekiben.

DISCUSSION QUESTIONS

1. Is fast food an effective method of mass feeding in an industrialized society?
2. Does the fast-food culture enhance or reduce food security?
3. What are the implications of the fast-food culture for future nutrition and health promotion efforts?
4. Discuss the pros and cons for airlines in attempting to reflect ethnic food cultures.
5. Why have Ekiben successfully preserved Japanese cultural food values?
6. Adduce and examine other examples of mass feeding from a bioculture point of view (e.g. street food).

References

CHAPTER 1

Abrahamsson, L. (1979) The Mothers Choice of Food for Herself and Her Baby, in *The Mother-Child Dyad: Dietary Aspects.*, Symposium of the Swedish Nutrition Foundation XIV, (ed. G. Blix), Almqvist & Wiksells, Uppsala, pp. 103–8.

Back, K.W. (1977) Food, Sex and Theory, in *Nutrition and Anthropology in Action,* (ed. T.K. Fitzgerald), Van Gorcum, Amsterdam, pp. 24–34.

Barnes, R.H. (1968) The Inseparability of Nutrition from the Social and Biological Sciences. *Nutrition et Dieta*, **10**, 1.

Bass, M.A., Wakefield, L.M. and Kolassa, K.M. (1979) *Community Nutrition and Individual Food Behavior,* Burgess Publishing, Minnesota.

Becker, M.H. (1974) The Health Belief Model and Personal Health Behavior. *Health Education Monograph*, **2**(4), 328–473.

Berkes, F. and Farkas, C.S. (1978) Eastern James Bay Cree Indians: Changing Patterns of Wild Food Use and Nutrition. *Ecol. Food & Nutr.*, **7**, 155–72.

Calnan, M. and Fieldhouse, P. (1986) Explaining variations in household food practices. Unpublished research.

Cattle, D.J. (1977) An Alternative to Nutritional Particularism, in *Nutrition and Anthropology in Action*, (ed. T.K. Fitzgerald), Van Gorcum, Amsterdam, pp. 35–45.

Committee on Food Habits (1945) *Manual for the Study of Food Habits,* NRC Bulletin 111, NAS, Washington, DC.

De Garine, I. (1970) The Social and Cultural Background of Food Habits in Developing Countries (Traditional Societies), in *Symposium on Food Cultism and Nutritional Quackery,* (ed. G. Blix), Swedish Nutrition Foundation, Almqvist & Wiksells, Uppsala. pp. 35–46.

DuBois, C. (1944) *The People of Alor: A Social-Psychological Study of an East Indian Island,* University of Minneapolis Press, Minneapolis.

Duhl, L.J. (1990) *The Social Entrepreneurship of Change,* Pace University Press, New York.

Eckstein, E.F. (1980) *Food, People and Nutrition,* AVI, Westport.

Fieldhouse, P. (1982) Nutrition and Education of the School Child. *World Rev. Nutr. & Diet.*, **40**, 83–112.

Fieldhouse, P. (1983) Behavioural Aspects of the Decision to Breastfeed. *Can. J. Home Ec.*, **32**(2), 88–93.

Fischer, L. (1950) *The Life of Mahatma Gandhi,* Harper & Row, New York.

Foster, G. (1962) *Traditional Cultures and the Impact of Technological Change,* Harper & Row, New York.

Freedman, R.L. (1977) Nutritional Anthropology: An Overview, in *Nutrition and Anthropology in Action,* (ed. T.K. Fitzgerald), Van Gorcum, Amsterdam, pp. 1–23.

Freedman, R.L. (1981) *Human Food Uses. A Cross-Cultural, Comprehensive Annotated Bibliography,* Greenwood Press, London.

Freedman, R.L. (1983) *Human Food Uses. A Cross-Cultural, Comprehensive Annotated Bibliography (Supplement)*, Greenwood Press, London.

Grivetti, L.E. and Pangborn, R.M. (1973) Food Habit Research: A Review of Approaches and Methods. *J. Nutr. Ed.*, **5**, 204–7.

Grivetti, L.E., Lamprecht, S.J., Rocke, H.J. and Waterman, A. (1987) Threads of Cultural Nutrition: Arts and Humanities. *Progress in Food and Nutrition Science*, **11**, 249–306.

Gussow, J.D. (1986) Women, food and the future, *J. Can. Diet. Assoc.*, **47**(3), 138–41.

Hanssen, M. (1980) The validity of the concept of health foods, in *Food and Health: Science and Technology*, (eds G.C. Birch and K.T. Parker), Applied Science Publishers, London, pp. 27–41.

Kahn, M. (1986) *Always hungry, never greedy: Food and the expression of hunger in a Melanesian society*, Cambridge University Press, Cambridge.

Khare, R.S. and Rao, M.S.A. (eds) (1986) *Food, Society, and Culture: Aspects in South Asian Food Systems*, Carolina Academic Press, Durham.

Krondl, M.M. and Boxen, G.G. (1975) Nutrition Behaviour, Food Resources and Energy, in *Gastronomy: The Anthropology of Food and Food Habits*, (ed. M. Arnott), Mouton Publishing, The Hague, pp. 113-120.

Kuhnlein, H. (1992) Dietary Change and Culture. *Ecology of Food and Nutrition*, **27**, 3–4.

Lewin, K. (1943) Forces Behind Food Habits and Methods of Change, in *The Problem of Changing Food Habits*, Bulletin No. 108, National Research Council, National Academy of Sciences, Washington, DC.

Lindenbaum, S. (1986) Rice and Wheat: The Meaning of Food in Bangladesh, in *Food, Society and Culture: Aspects in South Asian Food Systems*, (eds R.S. Khare and M.S.A. Rao), Carolina Academic Press, Durham, pp. 253–75.

Lowenberg, M.E., Todhunter, E.N. Wilson, E.D. Savage, J.R. and Lubawski, J.L.. (1979) *Food and People*, J. Wiley & Sons, New York, p. 129.

Maslow, A.H. (1970) *Motivation and Personality*, Harper & Row, New York.

May, J.M. (1957) The Geography of Food and Cooking. *Int. Record. Med.*, **170**, 231.

Mennel, S. (1985) *All Manners of Food*, Blackwell, Oxford.

Messer, E. (1984) Anthropological Perspectives on Diet. *Annu. Rev. Anthropol.*, **13**, 205–49.

Østbye, T., Pomerleau, J., White, M., Coolich, M and McWhinney, J. (1993) Food and Nutrition in Canadian 'Prime Time' Television Commercials. *Can. J. Public Health*, **84**(6), 370–4.

Pelto, G.H., and Jerome, N.W. (1978) Intracultural Diversity and Nutritional Anthropology, in *Health and the Human Condition: Perspectives on Medical Anthropology*, (eds M.H. Logan and E.E. Hunt), Duxbury Press, North Scituate, Massachusetts, pp. 222–8.

People's Food Commission, (1980) *The Land of Milk and Money*, Between The Lines, Kitchener, Ontario.

Rao, M.S.A. (1986) Conservatism and Change in Food Habits Among the Migrants in India: A Study in Gastrodynamics, in *Food, Society, and Culture: Aspects in South Asian Food Systems*, (eds R.S. Khare and M.S.A Rao), Carolina Academic Press, Durham, pp. 121–40.

Rogers, B. (1981) *The Domestication of Women*, Tavistock Publications, London.

Rogers, E.M. and Shoemaker, F.F. (1971) *Communication of Innovations*, Free Press, New York.

Rotberg, R.I. (1983) Nutrition and History. *Journal of Interdisciplinary History*, xiv(2), 199–534.

Rozin, P. (1990) Acquisition of Stable Food Preferences. *Nutr. Rev.*, **48**(2), 106–13.

Salisbury, H.E. (1969) *The 900 days – The Siege of Leningrad,* Harper & Row, New York.

Sanjur, D. (1982) *Social and Cultural Perspectives in Nutrition,* Prentice Hall, New Jersey.

Schaefer, O. and Steckle, J. (1980) *Dietary Habits of Native populations,* Science Advisory Board of the Northwest Territories.

Schaefer, O., Timmermans, J.F.W., Eaton, R.D.P. and Matthews, A.R. (1980) General and Nutritional Health in Two Eskimo Populations at Different Stages of Acculturation. *Can. J. Public Health,* **71**(6), 397–405.

Schlabach, J.H. (1991), *Extending the Table: A World Community Cookbook,* Herald Press, Scottdale, Pennsylvania.

Super, J.C. (1988) *Food, Conquest, and Colonization in Sixteenth-Century Spanish America,* UNM Press, Albuquerque.

Tylor, E.B. (1871) *Primitive Culture: Researches into the Development of Mythology, Philosophy, Religion, Language, Art and Custom,* J. Murray, London.

Uhle, A.F. and Grivetti, L.E. (1993) Alpine and Brazilian Swiss Food Patterns After a Century of Isolation. *Ecology of Food and Nutrition,* **29**, 119–38.

United States Department of Health and Human Services (1991) *Mass Media and Health: opportunities for improving the nations' health,* Office of Disease Prevention and Health Promotion, Washington, DC.

Wilson, C.S. (1973) Food Habits. A Selected Annotated Bibliography. *Journal of Nutrition Education,* 5(suppl.)

Wilson C.S. (1979) Food – Custom and Nurture. An annotated Bibliography on Sociocultural and Biocultural Aspects of Nutrition. *Journal of Nutrition Education,* **11**(suppl.).

CHAPTER 2

Back, K.W. (1977) Food, Sex and Theory, in *Nutrition and Anthropology in Action,* (ed. T.K. Fitzgerald), van Gorcum, Amsterdam, pp. 23–34.

Bass, M.A., Wakefield, L.M. and Kolasa, K.M. (1979) *Community Nutrition and Individual Food Behaviour,* Burgess Publishing, Minneapolis.

de Esquef, L. (1972) Dietary Habits of the Peasant of the Bolivian Highlands. *FAO Nutrition Newsletter,* **10**(2), 16–20.

de Garine, I.L. (1976) Food, Tradition and Prestige, in *Food, Man and Society,* (eds D. Walcher, N. Kretchmer and H.L. Barnett), Plenum Press, New York, pp. 150–73.

Eckstein, E.F. (1980) *Food, People and Nutrition,* AVI Publishing Co. Inc., Westport.

Grivetti, L.E. (1991a) Nutrition Past – Nutrition Today. Prescientific Origins of Nutrition and Dietetics. *Nutrition Today,* January/February, 13–24.

Grivetti, L.E. (1991b) Nutrition Past – Nutrition Today. Prescientific Origins of Nutrition and Dietetics. *Nutrition Today,* July/August, 18–29.

Grivetti, L.E. (1991c) Nutrition Past – Nutrition Today. Prescientific Origins of Nutrition and Dietetics. *Nutrition Today,* November/December, 6–17.

Grivetti, L.E. (1992) Nutrition Past – Nutrition Today. Prescientific Origins of Nutrition and Dietetics. *Nutrition Today,* May/June, 13–25.

Harwood, A. (1971) The Hot–Cold Theory of Disease. Implications for Treatment of Puerto Rican Patients. *JAMA,* **216,** 1153–8.

Hasan, K.A. (1971) The Hindu Dietary Practices and Culinary Rituals in a North Indian Village. *Ethnomedizin,* **1,** 43–70.

Jelliffe, D.B. (1967) Parallel Food Classification in Developing and Industrialised Countries. *Am. J. Clin. Nutr.,* **20,** 279–81.

Jelliffe, D.B. and Bennett, F.J. (1961) Cultural and Anthropological Factors in Infant Nutrition. *Fed. Proc.*, **20**(No.1 part 3), suppl. 7, 185–7.

Katona-Apte, J. (1977) The Socio-cultural Aspects of Food Avoidance in a Low Income Population in Tamilnad. *South India. J. Trop. Pediatr. Environ. Child Health*, **23**, 83–90.

Lindenbaum, S. (1986) Rice and Wheat: The Meaning of Food in Bangladesh, in *Food, Society, and Culture: Aspects in South Asian Food Systems*, (eds) R.S. Khare and M.S.A Rao, Carolina Academic Press, Durham, pp. 253–75.

Logan, M. (1972) Humoral Folk Medicine: A Potential Aid in Controlling Pellagra in Mexico. *Ethnomedizin*, **1**, 397–410.

McCracken, R.D. (1971) Lactase Deficiency: An Example of Dietary Evolution. *Current Anthropology*, **12**, 479–517.

Messer, E. (1984) Anthropological Perspectives on Diet. *Annu. Rev. Anthropol.*, **13**, 205–49.

Molony, C.H. (1975) Systematic Valence Coding of Mexican 'hot'-'cold' Food. *Ecol. Food. Nutr.*, **4**, 67–74.

Nash, O. (1968) *There's Always Another Windmill*, Little, Brown & Co., Boston.

Nichter, M. (1986) Modes of Food Classification and the Diet-Health Contingency: A South indian Case Study, in *Food, Society, and Culture: Aspects in South Asian Food Systems*, (eds R.S. Khare and M.S.A Rao), Carolina Academic Press, Durham, pp. 185–222.

Passim, H. and Bennett, J.W. (1943) *Social Process and Dietary Change*, National Research Council Bulletin 108, Washingon, DC.

Rao, M.S.A. (1986) Conservatism and Change in Food Habits Among the Migrants in India: A Study in Gastrodynamics, in *Food, Society, and Culture: Aspects in South Asian Food Systems*, (eds R.S. Khare and M.S.A Rao), Carolina Academic Press, Durham, pp. 121–40.

Rizvi, N. (1986) Food Categories in Bangladesh, and Its Relationship to Food Beliefs and Practices of Vulnerable Groups, in *Food, Society, and Culture: Aspects in South Asian Food Systems*, (eds R.S. Khare and M.S.A Rao), Carolina Academic Press, Durham, pp. 223–52.

Sanjur, D. (1974) Food Ideology Systems as Conditioners of Nutritional Practices. *Archivos Latinoamericanos de Nutricion*, **24**(1), Caracas, Venezuela.

Sanjur, D. (1982) *Social and Cultural Perspectives in Nutrition*, Prentice Hall, New Jersey.

Schutz, H.G., Rucker, M.H. and Russell, G.F. (1975) Food and Food Use Classification Systems. *Food Tech.*, **29**(3), 50–6, 60–4.

Yeung, D.L., Cheung, W.Y. and Sabry, J.H. (1973) The Hot–Cold Food Concept in Chinese Culture and its Application in a Canadian-Chinese Community. *J. Can. Diet. Assoc.*, **34**, 1–8.

CHAPTER 3

Ajayi, S.S. (1974) Giant Rat for meat and some taboos. *Oryx*, **1**, 379–80 (cited in Scoones *et al.*, 1992).

Bailey, C.T.P. (1927) *Knives and Forks*, Medici Society, London.

Balfet, H. (1976) Bread in Some Regions of the Mediterranean Area: A Contribution to the Studies on Eating Habits, in, *Gastronomy: the Anthropology of Food and Food Habits*, (ed. M. Arnott), Mouton Publishing, The Hague.

Barer-Stein, T. (1979) *You Eat What You Are*, McClelland & Stewart, Toronto.

Bornstein-Johanssen, A. (1976) Sorghum and Millet in Yemen, in *Gastronomy: The Anthropology of Food and Food Habits,* (ed. M. Arnott), Mouton Publishers, The Hague, pp. 287–95.

Campbell, M.L., Diamant, R.F. and Macpherson, B.D. (1992) *Dietary Survey of preschool children, women of child-bearing age and older adults in God's River, Nelson House and South Indian Lake,* Medical Services Branch, Health & Welfare Canada, Ottawa.

Crosby, A.W. Jr. (1972) *The Columbian Exchange: Biological and Cultural Consequences of 1492,* The Greenwood Press, Westport.

de la Reynière, G. (1968) *Almanach des Gourmands,* P. Waeffe.

Douglas, M. and Nicod, M. (1974) Taking the Biscuit: the Structure of British Meals. *New Society,* 19th December.

Dufour D.L. (1987) Insects as food; A case study from the northwest Amazon. *American Anthropologist,* **89,** 383–97.

Elias, N. (1978) *The Civilising Process,* Urizon Books, New York.

Farb, P. and Armelagos, G. (1980) *Consuming Passions: the Anthropology of Eating,* Houghton Mifflin Co., Boston.

Goldblith, S.A. (1992) The Legacy of Columbus, with Particular Reference to Foods. *Food Technology,* October, 62–85.

Goode, J., Curtis, K., and Theophano, J. (1984) A framework for the analysis of continuity and change in shared sociocultural rules for food use: The Italian-American pattern, in *Foodways as a Matrix of Regional and Ethnic Identity,* (eds L.K. Brown and K. Musell), University of Tennessee Press, Nashville, pp. 66–88.

Grandstaff, S.W. (1986) Trees in paddy fields in Northeast Thailand, in *Traditional Agriculture in Southeast Asia,* (ed. G. Marten), Westview Press, Boulder, Colorado, pp. 273-92.

Hanks, L.M. (1972) *Rice and Man: Agricultural Ecology in Southeast Asia,* Aldine-Atherton, Chicago.

Heiser, C.B. (1990) *Seed to Civilization,* Harvard University Press, Cambridge, Massachusetts.

Hunt, D. (ed.) (1992) *Native Indian Wild Game, Fish & Wild Foods Cookbook,* Fox Chapel Publishing, Lancaster, Pennsylvania.

Khare, R.S. (1986) The Indian Meal: Aspects of Cultural Economy and Food Use, in *Food, Society and Culture: Aspects in South Asian Food Systems,* (eds R.S. Khare and M.S.A. Rao), Carolina Academic Press, Durham, pp. 159–84.

Kyle, R. (1987) Rodents under the carving knife. *New Scientist,* **June,** 58–61.

Leach, Sir E. (1970) *Levi-Strauss,* Fontana, Glasgow.

Levi-Strauss, C. (1969) *The Raw and the Cooked,* Harper & Row, New York.

Mangelsdorf, P.C. (1978) (Original paper 1953) Wheat, in *Human Nutrition: Readings from Scientific American,* (eds N. Kretchmer and W. van B. Robertson), W.H.Freeman, San Francisco, pp. 70–9.

Markham, G. (1615) *The English Hus-Wife,* Roger Jackson, London.

Masefield, G.B., Wallis, M., Harrison, S.G. and Nicholson, B.E. (1969) *The Oxford Book of Food Plants,* Oxford University Press, Oxford.

Mennel, S. (1985) *All Manners of Food,* Blackwell, Oxford.

Mowat, F. (1965) *People of the Deer,* McClelland and Stewart Ltd., Toronto.

People of 'Ksan (1980), *Gathering What the Great Nature Provided,* Douglas & McIntyre, Vancouver.

Root, W. (1980) *Food. An authoritative and visual history and dictionary of the foods of the world,* Simon and Schuster, New York.

Rozin, E. (1992) *Blue Corn and Chocolate,* A.A. Knopf, New York.

References 239

Salaman, R.N. (1985) *The History and Social influence of the potato,* Cambridge University Press, Cambridge.

Schlabach, J.H. (1991) *Extending the Table. A World Community Cookbook,* Herald Press, Scottdale.

Scoones, I., Melnyk, M. and Pretty, J.N. (1992) *The Hidden Harvest: Wild Foods and Agricultural Systems. A literature review and annotated bibliography,* International Institute for Environment and Development (London); Swedish International Development Authority; World Wide Fund for Nature, London.

Simmonds, N.W. (ed.) (1976) *Evolution of Crop Plants,* Longman, London.

Taylor, K.D. (1968) An outbreak of rats in agricultural areas in Kenya in 1962. *East African Agriculture and Forestry Journal,* **34,** 66–77.

Thorne, J. Cuisine Mecanique, *Journal of Gastronomy,* Spring 1990.

Williams, B.J. (1973) *Evolution and Human Origins: an Introduction to Physical Anthropology,* Harper, New York.

Wilson, K.B. (1990) *Ecological Dynamics and Human Welfare: A case Study of Population, Health and Nutrition in Southern Zimbabwe,* PhD Thesis, Department of Anthropology, University College, London.

CHAPTER 4

Appadurai, A. (1981) Gastro-Politics in Hindu South Asia, *American Ethnologist,* **8,** 494–511.

Barer-Stein, T. (1979) *You Eat What You Are,* McClelland and Stewart, Toronto.

Bozak, G. (1973) Potlatch: Revival of a Lost Culture. *Performing Arts in Canada,* **10,** 14–16.

Clutesi, G. (1969) *Potlatch,* Morris Printing Co., Victoria.

Cohen, Y.A. (1961) Food and its Vicissitudes: A Cross-cultural Study of Sharing and Non-sharing, in *Social Structure and Personality,* (ed. Y.A. Cohen), Holt, Rinehart & Winston, New York, pp. 312–50.

Cohen, Y.A. (1968) Food Consumption Patterns, in *International Encyclopedia of the Social Sciences Vol 5,* (ed. D.L. Sills), MacMillan Co. & The Free Press, New York, pp. 508–13.

Cosman, M.P. (1981) *Medieval Holidays and Festivals,* Scribner, New York.

Crim, K., Bullard, R.A. and Shinn, L.D. (eds) (1981) *Abingdon Dictionary of Living Religions,* Abingdon, Nashville.

Cussler, M. and DeGive, M.L. (1952) *Twixt the Cup and the Lip: Psychological and Socio-cultural Factors Affecting Food Habits,* Twayne Publishing, New York.

de Garine, I.L. (1970) The Social and Cultural Background of Food Habits in Developing Countries (Traditional Societies), in *Symposium on Food Cultism and Nutritional Quackery,* (ed. G. Blix), Almqvist & Wiksells, Uppsala, pp. 34–46.

de Garine, I.L. (1976) Food, Tradition & Prestige, in *Food, Man and Society,* (eds D.N. Walcher, N. Kretchmer and H.L. Barnett), Plenum Press, New York, pp. 150–73.

de la Reynière, G. (1968) *Almanach des Gourmands,* P. Waeffe.

Douglas, M. (1972) Deciphering a meal, *Daedelus,* **101,** 61–81.

Drummond, J.C. and Wilbraham, A.(1957) *The Englishman's Food,* Revised edition, Jonathon Cape, London.

Dyson-Hudson, R. and Van Dusen, R. (1972) Food Sharing Among Young Children, *Ecol. Food & Nutr.,* **1,** 319–24.

Eckstein, E.F. (1980) *Food, People and Nutrition,* AVI Publishing Co. Inc., Westport.

Farb, P. and Armelagos, G. (1980) *Consuming Passions: the Anthropology of Eating,* Houghton Mifflin Co., Boston.

Firth, R. (1965) Offering and Sacrifice: Problems of Organisation, in *Reader in Comparative Religion: an Anthropological Approach,* (eds W.A. Lessa and E.Z. Vogt), Harper & Row, New York, pp. 185–94.

Firth, R. (1967) Themes in Economic Anthropology: A General Comment, in *Themes in Economic Anthropology,* (ed. R. Firth) A.S.A. Monographs No. 6, Tavistock, London, pp. 1–28.

Frazer, J.G. (1963) *The Golden Bough,* Abridged edition, Macmillan Publishing Co., New York.

Hardisty, D.L. (1977) *Ecological Anthropology,* J. Wiley & Son, New York.

Harris, M. (1974) *Cows, Pigs, Wars and Witches,* Random House, New York.

Harris, M. (1977) *Cannibals and Kings,* Random House, New York.

Harris, M.H. (1923) *A Thousand Years of Jewish History,* Bloch, New York.

Heiser, C.B. Jr. (1990) *Seed to Civilisation,* 2nd edn, W.H. Freeman & Co., San Francisco.

Hou, C. (1973) *To Potlatch or not to Potlatch,* British Columbia Teacher's Federation, Victoria.

Isaac, E. (1959) Influence of Religion on the Spread of Citrus. *Science,* **129,** 179–86.

Kahn, M. (1986) *Always hungry, never greedy: Food and the expression of hunger in a Melanesian society,* Cambridge University Press, Cambridge.

Katona-Apte, J. (1976) Dietary Aspects of Acculturation: Meals, Feasts and Fasts in a Minority Community in South Asia, in *Gastronomy: The Anthropology of Foods and Food Habits,* (ed. M. Arnott), Mouton Publishing, The Hague, pp. 315–26.

Khare, R.S. (1986) Hospitality, Charity and Rationing: Three Channels of Food Distribution in India, in *Food, Society and Culture: Aspects in South Asian Food Systems,* (eds R.S. Khare and M.S.A. Rao), Carolina Academic Press, Durham, pp. 277–96.

LaViolette, F.E. (1973) *The Struggle for Survival,* University of Toronto Pr., Toronto.

Lee, R.B. (1969) Eating Christmas in the Kalahari. *Natural History,* **78**(10), 14–22.

Mead, M. (1980) A Perspective on Food Patterns, in *Issues in Nutrition for the 1980's,* (eds L.A. Tobias and P.J. Thompson), Wadsworth Inc., Monterey, pp. 225–9.

Murphy, C.P.H. (1986) Piety and Honor: The Meaning of Muslim Feasts in Old Delphi, in *Food, Society and Culture: Aspects in South Asian Food Systems,* (eds R.S. Khare and M.S.A. Rao), Carolina Academic Press, Durham, pp. 89–119.

Packard, V. (1959) *The Status Seekers,* McKay, New York.

People of 'Ksan (1980), *Gathering What the Great Nature Provided,* Douglas & McIntyre, Vancouver.

Rodriguez, E.H. (1986) Kausay Huñuy: The Levelling Feast, Andenes; August–September. (cited in Schlabach, 1991).

Rohner, R.P. and Rohner, E.C. (1970) *The Kwakiutl Indians of British Columbia,* Holt, Rinehart & Winston, New York.

Schlabach, J.H. (1991) *Extending the Table. A World Community Cookbook,* Herald Press, Scottdale.

Schuchat, M.G. (1973) The School Lunch and its Cultural Environment, *J. Nutr. Ed.,* **5,** 116–18.

Simoons, F.J. (1961) *Eat Not This Flesh,* University of Wisconsin Press, Madison.

Smith, C.M. (1972) *Instant Status: or how to become a pillar of the Upper Middle Class,* Doubleday, New York.

Suttles, W. (1960) Affinal Ties, Subsistence and Prestige Among the Coast Salish, *Am. Anthrop.,* **62,** 296–305.

Tannahill, R. (1976) *Flesh and Blood*, Sphere Books, London.

Tylor, E.B. (1871) *Primitive Culture: Researches into the Development of Mythology, Religion, Language, Art and Custom*, J. Murray, London.

Young, M.W. (1971) *Fighting with Food: Leadership, Values and Social Control in a Massim Society*, Cambridge University Press, Cambridge.

CHAPTER 5

Bentley, A.L. (1992) *Eating for Victory: United States Food Rationing and the Politics of Domesticity during World War Two (World War II)*, PhD Thesis, University of Pennsylvania.

Bhatty, Z. (1980) *Economic Role and the Status of Women: A Case Study of Women in the Beedi Industry in Allahabad*, World Employment Programs Research Working Paper.

Calnan, M. and Fieldhouse, P. (1986) *Explaining Variations in Household Food Patterns* (unpublished research).

Charles N. and Kerr, M. (1988) *Women, food and families*, Manchester University Press, Manchester.

Coward, R. (1985) *Female Desires*, Grove Press, New York.

Dahlberg, F. (1981) *Woman the Gatherer*, Yale University Press, New Haven.

Delphy, C. (1979) Sharing the same table: the family and consumption, in *The Sociology of the Family: New Directions for Britain*, Sociological Review Monographs in the Family, Number 28, (ed. C.C. Harris), University of Keele, Keele, pp. 214–31.

Delphy, C. and Leonard, D. (1984) *The Family as as Economic System*, Paper presented to the Conference on the Institutionalisation of Sex Differences, University of Kent at Canterbury.

Eisenbraun, C.I. (1987) *The way to a man's heart is through his stomach*, Womens Studies Occasional Paper No. 6., University of Kent at Canterbury.

Gussow, J.D. (1986) Women, food and the future. *J. Can. Diet. Assoc.* 47(3), 138–41.

Gussow, J.D. (1987) The fragmentation of need: Women, food and marketing. Food is a feminist issue. *Heresies #21*, 6(1): 39–43.

Gussow, J.D. (1988) Does Cooking Pay? *J. Nutr. Ed.*, 20(5): 221–6.

Kahn, M. (1986) *Always hungry, never greedy: Food and the expression of hunger in a Melanesian society*, Cambridge University Press, Cambridge.

Kerr, M. and Charles, N. (1986) Servers and providers: the distribution of food within the family. *Sociol Rev.* 34(1), 115–57.

Maher, V. (1984) Work, Consumption and Authority Within the Household: A Moroccan Case Study, in *Of Marriage and the Market: Women's Subordination Internationally and Its Lessons*, (eds K. Young, C. Wolkowitz and R. McCullagh), Routledge and Kegan Paul, London, pp. 117–35.

Mead, M. (1976) Comments on the Division of Labour in Occupations Concerned with Food. *J. Am. Diet. Assoc.*, 68, 321–5.

Menchu, R. (1985) *I. Rigaberto Menchu: An Indian Woman in Guatemala*, Verso, London.

Mennel, S. (1985) *All Manners of Food*, Blackwell, Oxford.

Murcott, A. (1982) On the Social Significance of the Cooked Dinner in South Wales. *Soc. Sci. Inf.*, 21 (4/5).

Murdock, G.P. (1937) Comparative data on the division of labour by sex. *Social Forces*, 15(4): 551–3 (cited in Rogers, 1981, p. 15).

Murdock, G.P. and Provost, C. (1973) Factors in the division of labor by sex: a cross-cultural analysis. *Ethnology*, 12, 203–35.

Oakley, A (1974) *The Sociology of Housework,* Random House, New York.

Pyle, D. (1985) Indonesia: East Java Family Planning, Nutrition, and Income Generation Project, in *Gender Roles in Development Projects: A Case Book,* (eds C. Overholt, M.B, Anderson, K. Cloud and J.E. Austin), Kumarian Press, West Hartford, pp. 135–62.

Rogers, D. (1981) *The Domestication of Women,* Tavistock Publications, London.

Safilios-Rothschild, C. (1970) The Study of Family Power Structures: A Review 1960–69. *J. Marriage and the Family,* **32**(4), 681–98.

Sivard, R.L. (1985) *Women. A World Survey,* World Priorities, Washington, DC.

Twose, N. (1987) Africa's Precious Few. *New Internationalist,* October, p. 12.

Weismantel, M.J. (1988) *Food, Gender and Poverty in the Ecuadorian Andes,* University of Pennsylvania Press, Philadelphia.

WFDAC (1993) *The Hand That Feeds the World: Women's Role in Global Food Security,* World Food Day Association of Canada, Ottawa.

CHAPTER 6

Abdu'l-Baha. *Star of the West,* Vol IV, No. 18: 305.

Berman, L.A. (1982) *Vegetarianism and the Jewish Tradition,* Ktav Publishing, New York.

Bosley, G.C. and Hardinge, M.G. (1992) Seventh Day Adventists: Dietary Standards and Concerns, *Food Technology,* October, pp. 112–13.

Brown, J.C. (1963) *Understanding Other Cultures,* Prentice Hall, New Jersey.

Diener, P and Robkin, E.E. (1978) Ecology, Evolution, and the Search for Cultural Origins. *Curr. Anthrop.,* **19**, 493–540.

Douglas, M. (1970) *Purity and Danger: An Analysis of Concepts of Pollution and Taboo,* Penguin Books, Harmonsworth.

Farb, P. and Armelagos, G. (1980) *Consuming Passions: the Anthropology of Eating,* Houghton Mifflin Co., Boston.

Freidl, J. and Pfeiffer, J.E. (1977) *Anthropology: The Study of People,* Harpers College Press, New York.

Grivetti, L.E. (1980) Dietary Separation of Meat and Milk. A Cultural Geographical Inquiry, *Ecol. Food & Nutr.,* **9**, 203–17.

Grivetti, L.E. and Pangborn, R.M. (1974) Origin of Selected Old Testament Dietary Prohibitions., *J. Am. Diet. Assoc.,* **65**, 634–8.

Harris, M. (1977) *Cannibals and Kings,* Random House, New York.

Hornby, H. (1988) *Lights of Guidance: A Bahai Reference File,* Bahai Publishing Trust, New Delhi.

Kilara, A. and Iya, K.K. (1992) Food and Dietary Habits of the Hindu, *Food Technology,* October, pp. 94–104.

Misra, P.K. (1986) Food Among the Nomadic Gadulia Lohars, in *Food, Society, and Culture,* (eds R.S. Khare and M.S.A. Rao), Carolina Academic Press, Durham, pp. 141–58.

Murphy, C.P.H. (1986) Piety and Honour: The meaning of Muslim feasts in Old Delhi, in *Food, Society, and Culture,* (eds R.S. Khare and M.S.A. Rao), Carolina Academic Press, Durham, pp. 85–120.

People of 'Ksan (1980), *Gathering What the Great Nature Provided,* Douglas & McIntyre, Vancouver.

Pike (1992) The Church of Jesus Christ of Latter-day Saints: Dietary Practices and Health, *Food Technology,* October, pp. 118–21.

Regenstein, J.M. and Regenstein, C.E. (1992) The Kosher Food Market in the 1990s – A Legal View, *Food Technology,* October, pp. 122–6.

Sherman, S. (1991) The Passover Seder: Ritual Dynamics, Foodways, and Family Folklore, in *We Gather Together: Foods and Festival in American Life*, (eds T.C. and L.T. Humphrey), Ann Arbor: UMI Research Press, pp. 27–42.

Simoons, F.J. (1961) *Eat Not This Flesh*, University of Wisconsin Press, Madison.

Simoons, F.J. (1974) Fish as Forbidden Food: the Case of India, *Ecol. Food & Nutr.*, **3**, 184–201.

Tannahill, R. (1976) *Flesh and Blood*, Sphere Books, London.

All Biblical citations are from The New English Bible, Oxford University Press/Cambridge University Press, 1970.

CHAPTER 7

Aihara, H. (1985) *Basic Macrobiotics*, Japan Publications, Tokyo.

Berman, L.A. (1982) *Vegetarianism and the Jewish Tradition*, Ktav Publishing, New York.

Dagnelie, P.C and van Staveren, W.A. (1994) Macrobiotic nutrition and child health: results of a population-based, mixed longitudinal cohort study in The Netherlands, *Am. J. Clin. Nutr.*, **59**(suppl), S1187–96.

de Garine, I.L. (1970) The Social and Cultural Background of Food Habits in Developing Countries (Traditional Societies), in *Symposium on Food Cultism and Nutritional Quackery*, (ed. G. Blix), Almqvist & Wiksells, Uppsala, pp. 34–46.

Durning A.T. and Brough H.B. (1991) *Taking stock: animal farming and the environment*, Worldwatch Paper 103, Worldwatch Institute, Washington, DC.

Elias, N. (1978) *The Civilising Process*, Urizon Books, New York.

Gussow, J.D. (1994) Ecology and vegetarian considerations: does environmental responsibility demand the elimination of livestock?, *Am. J. Clin. Nutr.*, **59**(suppl), S1110–6.

Herbert, V. (1980) *Nutrition Cultism. Facts and Fictions*, George F. Stickley Co., Philadelphia.

Kandel, R.F. and Pelto, G.H. (1980) The Health Food Movement, in *Nutritional Anthropology*, (eds N.W. Jerome, R.F. Kandel & G.H. Pelto), Redgrave Publications, New York, pp. 327–63.

Kushi, M. (1985) *The Macrobiotic Way*, Avery Publishing Group Inc., New Jersey.

Mowbray, S. (1992) *The Food Fight: Truth, Myth and the Food-Health Connection*, Random House, Toronto.

Pugliese, M.T., Weyman-Daum, M.S., Moses,N. and Lifshitz, F. (1987) Parental Health Beliefs as a Cause of Nonorganic Failure to Thrive, *Pediatrics*, **80**(2), 175–82.

Rifkin, J. (1992) *Beyond beef: the rise and fall of the cattle culture*, Dutton, New York.

Robson, J.R.K., Konlande, J.E., Larkin, F.A., O'Connor, P.A. and Liu H-Y. (1974) Zen Macrobiotic dietary problems in infancy, *Pediatrics*, **53**, 326–9.

Singer, P. (1976) *Animal Liberation*, Jonathan Cape, London.

Singer, P. (1979) *Practical Ethics*, Cambridge University Press, London.

US Senate. Select Committee on Nutrition and Human Needs (1977) *Dietary Goals for the United States*, 2nd edn., Government Printing Office, Washington, DC.

Wang, V.L. (1971) Food Information of Homemakers and 4-H Youths, *J. Am. Diet. Assoc.*, **58**, 215.

Whorton, J.C. (1994) Historical development of vegetarianism, *Am. J. Clin. Nutr.*, **59**(suppl): S1103–9.

Young, J.H. (1970) Historical Aspects of Food Cultism and Nutrition Quackery, in *Symposium on Food Cultism and Nutritional Quackery*, (ed. G. Blix), Swedish Nutritional Foundation, Almqvist & Wiksells, Uppsala, pp. 9–21.

CHAPTER 8

Arens, W. (1979) *The Man-Eating Myth: Anthropology and Anthrophagy*, Oxford University Press, New York.
Bolton, J.M. (1972) Food Taboos Among The Orang Asli in West Malaysia: A Potential Nutritional Hazard, *Am. J. Clin. Nutr.*, **25**, 789–99.
Bringeus, N.A. (1975) Food and Folk Beliefs: On Boiling Blood Sausage, in *Gastronomy: the Anthropology of Food and Food Habits*, (ed. M. Arnott), Mouton Publishing, The Hague.
Brown, W.N. (1957) The Sanctity of the Cow in Hinduism. *The Madras University Journal*, **28**, 29–49 (cited in Lodrick, 1981.)
Cohen, Y.A. (1968) Food Consumption Patterns, in *International Encyclopedia of the Social Sciences*, Vol. 5, (ed. D.L. Sills), MacMillan Co. & The Free Press, New York, pp. 508–13.
de Garine, I.L. (1970) The Social and Cultural Background of Food Habits in Developing Countries (Traditional Societies), in *Symposium on Food Cultism and Nutritional Quackery*, (ed. G. Blix), Swedish Nutritional Foundation, Almqvist & Wiksells, Uppsala, pp. 34–46.
de Garine, I.L. (1976) Food, Tradition and Prestige, in *Food, Man and Society*, (eds D.N. Walcher, N. Kretchmer and H.L. Barnett), Plenum Press, New York, pp. 150–73.
Diener, P., Nonini, D. and Robkin, E.E. (1978) The Dialectics of the Sacred Cow: Ecological Adaptation vs. Political Appropriation in the Origins of India's Cattle Complex. *Dialectical Anthropology*, **3**(3), 221–41.
Farb, P. and Armelagos, G. (1980) *Consuming Passions: The Anthropology of Eating*, Houghton Mifflin, Boston.
Ferro-Luzzi, G.E. (1974) Food Avoidances During the Puerperium and Lactation in Tamilnad. *Ecol. Food & Nutr.*, **3**, 7–15.
Freidl, J. and Pfeiffer, J.E. (1977) *Anthropology: The Study of People*, Harpers College Press, New York.
Gade, D.W. (1976) Horsemeat as Human Food in France. *Ecol. Food & Nutr.*, **5**, 1–11.
Harris, M. (1965) The Myth of the Sacred Cow, in *Man, Culture and Animals*, (eds A. Leeds and A.P. Vayda), American Association for the Advancement of Science, Publication No. 78, Washington, DC, pp. 217–28.
Harris, M. (1974) *Cows, Pigs, Wars and Witches*, Random House, New York.
Harris, M. (1978) India's Sacred Cow. *Human Nature*, **1**(2), 28–36.
Hogg, G. (1961) *Cannibalism and Human Sacrifice*, Pan Books, London.
Holt, V.M. (1885) *Why Not Eat Insects?* E.W. Classey Ltd., Middlesex (reprinted 1969).
Hope, M. (1975) Food Taboos and Nutrition in the Caribbean. *Cajanus*, **8**, 190–3.
Jelliffe, D.B. and Jelliffe, E.F.P. (1978) Food Habits and Taboos: How Have They Protected Man in His Evolution? *Prog. Human Nutr.*. **2**, 67–76.
Kahn, M. (1986) *Always hungry, never greedy: Food and the expression of hunger in a Melanesian society*, Cambridge Universtity Press, Cambridge.
Leach, E.R. (1976) *Culture and Communications: The Logic by which Symbols are connected*, Cambridge University Press, Cambridge.
Leach, M. (1972) *Standard Dictionary of Folklore*, Funk & Wagnalls, New York.

Lewis, I.M. (1986) *Religion in Context: Cults and Charisma*, Cambridge University Press, New York.

Lindenbaum, S. (1977) The Last Course: Nutrition and Anthropology in Asia, in *Nutrition and Anthropology in Action*, (ed. T.K. Fitzgerald), van Gorcum, Amsterdam.

Lodrick, D.O. (1981) *Sacred Cows, Sacred Places*, University of California Press, Berkeley.

Malinowski, B. (1963) *Sex, Culture and Myth*, R. Hart-Davis, London.

Newman, L.F. (1969) Folklore of Pregnancy: Wives Tales in Contra Costa County, California. *West. Folklore*, **28**, 112–35.

Odend'hal, S. (1972) Gross Energetic Efficiency of Indian Cattle in Their Environment. *J. Human Ecol.*, **1**, 1–27.

Ogbeide, O. (1974) Nutritional Hazards of Food Taboos and Preferences in Mid West Nigeria. *Am. J. Clin. Nutr.*, **27**, 213–16.

Pariser, E.R. and Hammerle, O.A. (1966) Some Cultural and Economic Limitations on the Use of Fish as Food. *Food Tech.*, **20**(5), 61–4.

People of 'Ksan (1980), *Gathering What the Great Nature Provided*, Douglas & McIntyre, Vancouver.

Read, P.P. (1974) *Alive*, J.P. Lippincott Co., New York.

Shifflett, P.A. (1976) Folklore and Food Habits, *J. Am. Diet. Assoc.*, **68**, 347–50.

Shifflett, P.A. and Nyberg, K.L. (1978) Toward a social psychology of food use. *Mid-American Review of Sociology*, 3(2), 35–54.

Simoons, F.J. (1961) *Eat Not This Flesh*, University of Wisconsin Press, Madison.

Simoons, F.J. (1979) Questions in the Sacred Cow Controversy. *Current Anthropology*, **20**, 467–93.

Srinivasan, D. (1979) *Concept of Cow in the Rigveda*, Motilal Banarsidass, Delhi.

Taylor, R.L. (1973) *Butterflies in my Stomach: Insects in Human Nutrition*, Woodbridge Press Publishing Co., Santa Barbara.

Trant, H. (1954) Food Taboos in East Africa. *Lancet*, **2**, 703–5.

Wilson, C.S. (1973) Food Taboos of Childbirth: The Malay example. *Ecol. Food & Nutr.*, **2**, 267–74.

Wodehouse, P.G. (1957) *Very Good, Jeeves!* Penguin, Middlesex (reprinted1978).

Yalman, N. (1967) *Under the Bo Tree: Studies in Caste, Kinship and Marriage in the Interior of Ceylon*, University of California Press, Berkeley.

CHAPTER 9

Agras, S.W., Berkowitz, I.R., Hammer, L.C. and Kraemer, H.C. (1988) Relationships between the eating behaviors of parents and their 18-month-old children: a laboratory study. *Int. J. Eating Disorders*, **7**, 461–8.

Birch, L.L. (1992) Children's Preferences for High-Fat Foods. *Nutr. Rev.*, **50**(9), 249–55.

Bruch, H. (1974) *Eating Disorders. Obesity, Anorexia Nervosa and the Person Within*, Routledge & Kegan Paul, London.

Cohen, Y.A. (1961) Food and its Vicissitudes: a Cross-cultural Study of Sharing and Non-sharing, in *Social Structure and Personality*, (ed. Y.A. Cohen), Holt, Rinehart & Winston, New York, pp. 312–50.

Davis, C.M. (1928) Self-selection of Diets by Newly Weaned Infants: an Experimental Study. *Am. J. Dis. Child.*, **36**, 651–79.

Davis, C.M. (1939) Results of the Self-selection of Diets by Young Children. *Can. Med. Assoc. J.*, **41**, 257–61.

Dickens, G. and Trethowan, W.H. (1971) Cravings and Aversions During Pregnancy. *J. Psychosomat. Res.*, **15**, 259–68.

Dickins, D. and Ford, R.N. (1942) Geophagy (dirt eating) Among Mississippi Negro Schoolchildren. *Am. Sociol. Rev.*, **7**, 59–65.

Eastwell, H.D. (1979) A Pica Epidemic: A price for sedentarism among Australian Ex-Hunter-Gatherers. *Psychiatry*, **42**(3), 264–73.

Garb, J.L. and Stunkard, A.J. (1974) Taste Aversions in Man. *Am. J. Psychiatry*, **13**, 1204–7.

Gifft, H.H., Washbon, M.B. and Harrison, G.G. (1972) *Nutrition, Behaviour and Change*, Prentice Hall, New Jersey.

Hochstein, G. (1968) Pica: A Study in Medical and Anthropological Explanation, in *Essays on Medical Anthropology*, (ed. T. Weaver), Southern Anthropological Society Proceedings No.1, pp. 88–97.

Hook, E.B. (1978) Dietary Cravings and Aversions During Pregnancy. *Am. J. Clin. Nutr.*, **31**, 1355–62.

Hunter, J.M. (1973) Geophagy in Africa and the United States: A Culture-Nutrition Hypothesis. *Geog. Rev.*, **63**, 170–95.

Klesges, R.C., Stein, R.J., Eck, L.H., Isbell, T.R. and Klesges, L.M. (1991) Parental influence on food selection in young children and its relationship to childhood obesity. *Am. J. Clin. Nutr.*, **53**, 859–64.

Korslund, M.K. and Eppright, E.S. (1967) Taste Sensitivity and Eating Behaviour of Preschool Children. *J. Home Economics*, **59**, 168–71.

Moore, H.B. (1952) Psychologic Facts and Dietary Fancies. *J. Am. Diet. Assoc.*, **28**, 789–94.

Murray, H.L. and Watson, R.H.J. (1978) Personality and Food Preference. *Proc. Nutr. Soc.*, **37**, 36A.

Orbach, S. (1978) *Fat is a Feminist Issue*, Paddington Press, New York and London.

Pangborn, R.M. (1975) Cross-cultural Aspects of Flavour Preference. *Food Tech.*, **29**(6), 34–6.

Perimenis, L. (1991) The Ritual of Anorexia Nervosa in Cultural Context. *J. Am. Cult.*, **14**(4), 48–59.

Pilgrim, F.J. (1957) The Components of Food Acceptance and their Measurement. *Am. J. Clin. Nutr.*, **5**, 171–5.

Pilgrim, F.J. (1961) What Foods do People Accept or Reject?, *J. Am. Diet. Assoc.*, **38**, 439–43.

Pope, J.F., Skinner, J.D. and Carruth, B.R. (1992) Cravings and aversions of pregnant adolescents. *J. Am. Diet. Assoc.*, **92**(12), 1479–82.

Rozin, P. (1978) The Use of Characteristic Flavourings in Human Culinary Practice, in *Flavor: Its Chemical, Behavioral and Commercial Aspects*, (ed. C.M. Apt), Westview Press, Colorado, pp. 101–27.

Rozin, P. (1990) Acquisition of Stable Food Preferences. *Nutr. Rev.*, **48**(2), 106–13.

Shack, W. (1971) Hunger, Anxiety and Ritual: Deprivation and Spirit Possession among the Gurage of Ethiopa. *Man*, **6**, 30–43.

Snow, L.F. and Johnson, S.M. (1978) Folklore, Food, Female Reproductive Cycle. *Ecol. Food Nutr.*, **7**, 41–9.

Solien, N.L.A. (1954) A Cultural Explanation of Geophagy. *Florida Anthrop.*, **7**, 1–9.

Story, M. and Brown, J.E. (1987) Do young children instinctively know what to eat? The studies of Clara Davis revisited. *N. Engl. J. Med.*, **316**(2), 103–6.

Vermeer, D.E. (1966) Geophagy Among the Tiv of Nigeria. *Assn. Am. Geog. Ann.*, **56**, 197–204.

Vermeer, D.E. (1971) Geophagy Among the Ewe of Ghana. *Ethnology*, **10**, 56–72.

Vermeer, D.E. and Frate, D.A. (1975) Geophagy in a Mississippi County. *Assn. Am. Geog. Ann.*, **65**, 414–24.

Weinberg, J. (1972) Psychologic Implications of the Nutritional Needs of the Elderly. *J. Am. Diet. Assoc.*, **60**, 293–6.

CHAPTER 10

Aviation Week and Space Technology (1993), July 19, p. 15.

Jacobsen, M.F. and Fritschner, S. (1991), *Fast Food Guide*, Workman Publishing, New York.

Kamekura, J., Bosker, G. and Watanabe, M. (1989) *Ekiben: the art of the Japanese Box lunch*, Chronicle Books, San Francisco.

Kodansha (ed.) (1991) *Oishii Ekiben Hudoki*, Kodansha Culture Books, Japan.

Love, J.F. (1986) *Behind the Arches*, Bantam, New York.

Ritzer, G. (1993) *The McDonaldization of Society*, Pine Forge Press, Newbury Park.

Terzani, A. and Wolf, R (1987) *Japan: the beauty of food*, Rizzoli, New York.

Index